Praise for Dr. Morris and *THE WELLNESS CODE*

"In *The Wellness Code*, Dr. Morris achieves what few have done. He not only explains why diet fads, exercise gimmicks, and quick fixes are NOT the answer, but he also provides scientific, yet understandable, explanations of what CAN be the answer to years of wellness ahead. Even for those who are set in their lifestyle, Dr. Morris provides feasible methods of breaking into a better way of living so that we can all live long and prosper."

> —NINA SHAPIRO, M.D., Bestselling Author of *Take a Deep Breath: Clear the Air for the Health of Your Child* and Professor, Department of Head and Neck Surgery, David Geffen School of Medicine at UCLA

"Like most of us, I am able to start and get successful early results from a diet. Then slowly it slips away. Why? In reading *The Wellness Code* I learned why and it was eye-opening. Thank you, Dr. Morris for a clear and well thought out long-term plan for healthy change."

> —JORDAN KERNER, Producer of *Charlotte's Web*, *Fried Green Tomatoes*, *The Smurfs*, and *The Mighty Ducks*

"Dr. Brian Morris is a tremendously caring physician who exemplifies all that is inspiring about being a doctor. He is a compassionate and humble human being who prioritizes his patients' well-being above anything else. Everyone who reads *The Wellness Code* will be motivated to live a happy and healthy life."

> —JEFFREY PUGLISI, M.D., Glenville Medical Concierge Care, Greenwich, CT and President of the Greenwich Medical Society

"*The Wellness Code* is a true game-changer. It is required reading for anyone looking to finally lose the weight and make a health transformation."

> —GAVIN JAMES, President and CEO, Western Asset Mortgage Capital

"*The Wellness Code* is the only "diet" book you will ever need to read. Dr. Morris will show you how to finally lose those pounds."

> —PAR CHADHA, Chairman and CEO, HGM Fund

"Wait!!! If you read and absorb *The Wellness Code*, you will never be the same. This book is a treasure that has the power to change your life forever. Dr. Morris has spent decades learning and teaching the correct balance of nutritional, physical and spiritual well-being. Recalibrate your habits and use the treasured wisdom of this book to reach your maximum potential in every aspect of life."

—PASTOR DUDLEY C. RUTHERFORD, Bestselling Author of *God Has an App for That: Discover God's Solutions for the Major Issues of Life*

"For anyone who is about to begin a transformation of their body, this book is required reading as it contains all the ingredients to achieve that success!"

—MICHAEL RAY, CEO, ProSource Insights and President and CEO, Focus of Greater Los Angeles

"Dr. Morris has created a health resource that will stand the test of time. *The Wellness Code* truly changed my life."

—CYRUS BARAGHOUSH, Director of Patient and Guest Services, UCLA Heath

"In *The Wellness Code,* Dr. Morris offers a comprehensive strategy for transforming your relationship with food, your body, and your health. The weight loss and wellness tools are practical, manageable, and sustainable. Dr. Morris lays out the interconnectedness of nutrition to other habits such as exercise, sleep, and stress. The focus is on eating the correct amounts and types of food, forming healthy habits, and constructing your environment to support optimal eating. This is a recipe for long-term success."

—CYNTHIA SASS, M.P.H., M.A., R.D., C.S.S.D., Nutritionist and New York Times Bestselling Author

"Dr. Brian Morris is a dedicated preventive medicine physician who distills his experience into a valuable science-based program for enhancing total wellness."

—DAVID HEBER, M.D., Ph.D., Professor Emeritus of Medicine and Public Health and Founding Director, UCLA Center for Human Nutrition, David Geffen School of Medicine at UCLA and Bestselling Author of *What Color Is Your Diet?*

"What makes *The Wellness Code* special is its emphasis on long-lasting, life-changing habits, rather than quick fixes that too often fail. There's no doubt that Dr. Morris's book can profoundly transform your life. I highly recommend it."

—TODD THIBAUD, Singer-Songwriter, Guitarist, and Former Lead Singer of The Courage Brothers

"*The Wellness Code* is a beautiful holistic merging of modern paradigm and ancient wisdom."

—RABBI IRA ROSENFELD, Co-Founder of Or Echad and HomeShul, Los Angeles, CA

"Dr. Morris has developed a very thorough wellness program that is ideal for busy executives and professionals at all levels. I thoroughly recommend his wellness program and approach."

—MOHAN MAHESWARAN, President and CEO, Semtech Corporation

"*The Wellness Code* is a practical approach to a healthier lifestyle. If we follow his advice we will be able to enjoy the benefits of long lasting changes in our lives. A truly useful read."

—LAURENT DEGRYSE, Chairman of the Board, Soft Kinetic, Managing Partner, Hunza Management

"Alas! *The Wellness Code* is NOT another warmed over repackaged, updated version of last year's model of the pursuit of health and happiness. Dr. Morris has written a prophetic "new thing" in the ongoing battle of the bulge and blues by finding common ground between the spiritual and existential dimensions of mind, body, and spirit. This is the rare book that synthesizes profound principles and traditional truths into practical paths of achievable success. *The Wellness Code* is chock-full of innovative approaches and creative strategies that will put you on a path to a new dimension of health."

—BISHOP KENNETH C. ULMER, Ph.D., Bestselling Author of *Knowing God's Voice: Learn How to Hear God Above the Chaos of Life and Respond Passionately in Faith* and Vice Chair of the Board, The King's University.

"*The Wellness Code* is advice for your body and mind based on real science instead of fads or theories. You will live better and healthier with this book."

"Dr. Morris is an extraordinary physician whose acumen and care benefit his patients immeasurably. *The Wellness Code* increases the reach of his incredible program for health and living."

The

WELLNESS CODE

The WELLNESS CODE

The Evidence-Based Prescription for
Weight Loss, Longevity, Health, and Happiness

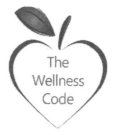

BRIAN MORRIS, M.D.

Vista Hill Press
A Division of Five Minute Network, LLC
Los Angeles

THE WELLNESS CODE:
The Evidence-Based Prescription for Weight Loss, Longevity, Health and Happiness

Copyright © 2015 by Brian Morris, M.D.

Published by
Vista Hill Press
A Division of Five Minute Network, LLC
907 Westwood Blvd., Suite 405
Los Angeles, CA 90024

First Edition: 2015

Cover design by Bojan Rekovic
Logo design by Arielle Morris
Book Layout by Nat Mara

Library of Congress Cataloging-in-Publication Data is available

ISBN-13: 978-0-9968377-0-5

For Rebecca, Arielle, Eliana, Avigail, and Jacob—
my family, who taught me the meaning of love.

Contents

Introduction   *1*

Chapter 1: The Story of The Wellness Code   5

Chapter 2: Why The Wellness Code Works and Diets Don't   13

    Small Changes vs. Big Changes   14
    Information Isn't Enough   16
    Tunnel Vision   17
    Stages of Change   18
    One You vs. Two You's   22
    The Four-Legged Stool of Wellness   24

Chapter 3: The Wellness Mindset   29

    Character Trait 1: Personal Responsibility   30
    Character Trait 2: Prioritization   31
    Character Trait 3: Self-Discipline   32
    Character Trait 4: Realism   33
    Character Trait 5: Do The Right Thing   34
    Character Trait 6: Self-Respect   36
    Character Trait 7: Perseverance   37

Chapter 4: The Three Steps to Habit Building   38

Chapter 5: The Seven Tools for Living The Wellness Code   42

Chapter 6: The Wellness Code   51

    Nutrition   53

        Habit 1:   Eat the Correct Number of Calories   54
        Habit 2:   Eat the Correct Types of Calories   57
        Habit 3:   Downsize Your Eating Habits   64
        Habit 4:   The ADAPT Process   66

Habit 5: Eat Before You Eat   68

Habit 6: Make Healthy Food Convenient   71

Habit 7: Eat Breakfast   74

Habit 8: Read the Label   76

Habit 9: Guide to Healthy Restaurant Eating   80

Habit 10: Prepare Your Own Food   85

Habit 11: Eat the Clean Calories   87

Habit 12: Weigh Yourself Regularly   92

Habit 13: Automate Eating   93

Habit 14: Slow Down   95

Habit 15: Avoid Excessive Alcohol   97

Exercise   99

Habit 16: Practice Regular Physical Activity   100

Habit 17: The Importance of Aerobic Exercise   103

Habit 18: Weight Training   106

Habit 19: Stretch   108

Habit 20: Meditate   110

Personal   115

Habit 21: Plan Your Calendar Weekly   116

Habit 22: Practice Good Dental Hygiene   119

Habit 23: Practice Safe Driving Habits   122

Habit 24: Anticipation   125

Habit 25: Do Not Smoke   129

Habit 26: Sleep Well   131

Habit 27: Allergy-Proof Yourself and Your Environment   135

Habit 28: Find Joy   139

Habit 29: Practice Hobbies   141

Habit 30: Simplify Your Life   144

Habit 31: Take a Break   149

Habit 32: Read Every Day   151

Social   153

Habit 33: Volunteer Each Week   154

Habit 34: Love Your Self   156

Habit 35:   Love Your Spouse or Partner   158
Habit 36:   Love Your Children   161
Habit 37:   Love Your Friends & Family   164
Habit 38:   Participate in Your Community   166
Habit 39:   Find Mentors   170

Spirituality and Values   175

Habit 40:   Live Your Values   176
Habit 41:   Practice Your Faith or Spiritual Practice   178
Habit 42:   Let Go of Emotional Pain from the Past   180
Habit 43:   Live Within Your Means   184
Habit 44:   Practice Integrity   186
Habit 45:   Leave a Legacy   188
Habit 46:   Visualize Before You Act   191
Habit 47:   Practice Gratitude: The Secret to Happiness   194
Habit 48:   The Power of Music   204
Habit 49:   Forgiveness   209
Habit 50:   Practice Mindfulness   213

Chapter 7: Conclusion: Living The Wellness Code   217

Acknowledgements   221
Scientific Reference Articles and Suggested Readings   223
Tables   263
Index   269

Introduction

Living a healthy lifestyle should be simple. You know what to do to be healthy: eat sensibly, exercise consistently, get a good night's sleep, and avoid excessive stress. It seems simple enough. Well, simple doesn't mean that it's easy because most of the patients that I see at UCLA struggle to practice a healthy lifestyle. And, since two out of three Americans are overweight or obese, maintaining a healthy lifestyle is clearly a challenge for the majority of us.

This is why I've spent over two decades of medical practice creating a process that has helped thousands of my patients achieve a healthy lifestyle. I call this process *The Wellness Code* and it has become both my passion and my mission as a physician.

True mastery of wellness involves both understanding and practicing the habits of healthy living. In other words, you need to know both *what to do* and *how to do it.* Thus, *The Wellness Code* combines the knowledge of what is needed for optimal wellness with the practical information needed to implement a healthy lifestyle.

Why do I call this a code? The word "code" generally has two definitions. A "code" can be a system of letters, numbers, sounds, or other symbols that provide access to something important. However, "code" can also have a second meaning. A code can be a way of life; a set of principles for how you live each day. My hope is that "The Wellness Code" will serve both of these purposes by providing access to a system for lifelong optimal health and happiness.

My patients tell me that *The Wellness Code* is unlike anything they've read or heard before. I believe that's because the focus of *The Wellness Code* is on practical strategies and tools that work for long-term success. This is not another diet program that offers short-term results and long-term pain. Instead, this program offers practical solutions that can last a lifetime.

The Wellness Code isn't a diet. It's a way of life.

A major problem with most diet and lifestyle programs is that they don't take into account how people change. Most diets approach a healthy lifestyle with the mistaken belief that people can immediately rework their life all at once. This simply isn't the way that life works. When these well-intentioned diet programs recommend that you immediately implement their entire system, it is generally a set-up for failure. Even if you are successful in making such sweeping changes, it is unlikely that you will be able to maintain these changes over the long-term.

Another reason most diets are unsuccessful is that they provide the information needed to be healthy, but don't provide the tools needed to actually implement this knowledge. There is a big difference between theoretically knowing what to do and actually living these practices on a daily basis. Just as listening to music for years doesn't qualify you to perform a concert at Madison Square Garden, simply reading about the practice of healthy living doesn't prepare you to live a healthy lifestyle. I believe the disconnection between knowing and doing is the root cause of most people's health struggles. *The Wellness Code*, on the other hand, teaches a process in which you learn both what you need to do for optimal wellness and also how to implement these practices.

Within this book, I've included a wealth of information about the "what to do," as well as the "how to do it" for the practice of wellness. You will notice that I repeat some of the important principles throughout the different sections of the book. This is intentional. Some of you will read this book from cover to cover while others will only read the sections that are of interest. I've written this book so that it can be read either way.

Before we get into the nuts and bolts of *The Wellness Code*, let's define what I mean by "wellness." The traditional definition of wellness is "the state or condition of good physical and mental health." For me, that's an incomplete definition as it only includes part of how I define wellness. Do you remember the original television show *Star Trek*? Leonard Nimoy played Spock on that show and would sometimes say a catch phrase that perfectly encapsulates what I believe is true wellness: "Live long and prosper." Mr. Spock realized there are actually two components to wellness:

1. Optimal health (to prosper)
2. Longevity (to live long)

The first component of wellness is to have optimal health—to live a good, healthy life rich with depth and fulfillment, optimal health, and meaningful relationships. The second key to wellness is longevity. You want to live a life full of great experiences, great relationships, and great physical and mental health, but you also want to hang around for a long while. When I talk about trying to achieve wellness, I mean that you're striving for both a healthy and long life. Living a life of wellness involves living a healthy, vibrant life so that you can savor your precious moments with friends, family and your community.

In addition to Spock's message, I would go a step further and add one more component to the definition of wellness. That third component of wellness is happiness. By happiness, I don't mean the sort of temporary feeling that passes in an hour or a day. I'm referring to a deep rooted appreciation and fulfillment in life. It is this joy in life, when combined with health and longevity, which leads us down the road to true wellness. Thus, my definition of wellness includes all three components: longevity, health and happiness.

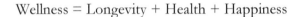

Wellness = Longevity + Health + Happiness

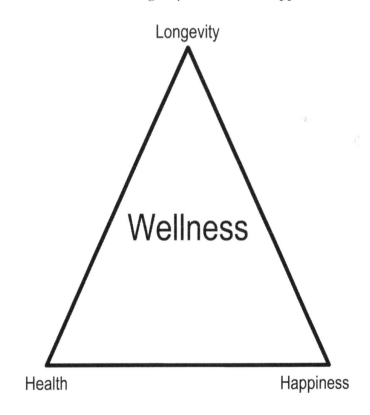

Throughout this book, when I mention wellness, feel free to mentally substitute "living long, living well, and living happily." If there's a "secret" to *The Wellness Code*, it is to master the habits of these three arenas: longevity, health and happiness.

The Wellness Code is a practical roadmap to help you master longevity, health, and happiness in a way that will last a lifetime. This book will provide you with the information necessary to achieve optimal wellness. In addition, I will walk you through *how* to incorporate this information into your day-to-day life in a way that will last.

By practicing *The Wellness Code*, you will learn the strategies that have worked for my patients to find optimal health and longevity while still living their busy and demanding lives. And we're going to have some fun along the way as well! So, let's get started by going back to 1998 when the idea for this book was hatched.

CHAPTER 1:

The Story of The Wellness Code

The story of this book began on February 21, 1998 when I had what I call my Jerry Maguire moment. Remember the scene in that great Tom Cruise movie when Jerry Maguire has his "*eureka*" moment where he's inspired to write the mission statement that completely changes his life? We all have those moments in our lives when a flash of clarity changes us forever.

I had just started my first medical practice and was extremely busy. Even though I've always prided myself on being in excellent physical condition, I was unfortunately ignoring my health. I knew how to take good care of myself, but I was working very long hours and was living off takeout food and getting far too little exercise.

That winter, I wanted a break from the bitter Boston weather so I flew down to South Florida to visit my Grandma Emma in West Palm Beach. I figured it would be a nice respite of golf, sun and pampering from my loving grandmother.

When I arrived at Grandma Emma's condo, the first thing she said to me was, "Brian, wow! You've gotten fat!" It was painful to hear my grandmother say that to my face. However, I could always count on Grandma Emma for her blunt honesty. I immediately ran to the mirror, looked at myself and realized that she was right. A tennis player for most of my life, I had always been in great shape and weight had never been an issue for me. Because I was so busy starting my professional life, I hadn't noticed that I had gradually gained about twenty pounds. Grandma Emma sure noticed.

At first, I was hurt. How could my grandmother say such a thing to me? Then I became angry at myself for letting this happen. After four years of medical school, three years of internal medicine residency training, and several years of medical practice, I knew a lot better. Despite all of that, I found myself heading down the path of weight gain due to poor lifestyle choices which could eventually lead to high blood pressure, high cholesterol, diabetes, heart disease, and even cancer if things didn't change.

Once I got over my bruised feelings, I started to come to terms with the difficult realization that I needed to learn how to actually live a healthy lifestyle. I already knew what foods to eat, how to exercise, how much sleep I needed, and how to control stress. However, despite having an intellectual understanding of how to be healthy, I wasn't practicing these habits on a consistent basis. I wasn't walking the walk. I saw this mirrored in the patients I was seeing at the office and in the hospital as well. The vast majority of my patients knew exactly what they should be doing, but were not living in a manner consistent with that knowledge.

Let me suggest that we've reached a point in our society where most of us know what we're supposed to do to be healthy. We're supposed to eat healthy foods such as fruits and vegetables, lean protein sources, and healthy fats in reasonable portions. We're supposed to exercise regularly. We're supposed to get a good night's sleep each night. We're supposed to avoid excessive stress. Sound familiar? You've probably heard all this before.

Well, despite knowing all that, today approximately two-thirds of all Americans are either overweight or obese. Yes, you read that correctly: only one in three Americans is in the "normal" weight range. And, because of poor lifestyle habits, the incidence of high blood pressure, diabetes, autoimmune diseases, and many cancers are skyrocketing. Sadly, we're witnessing a health crisis of epic proportions.

Genetics do play a role in this equation—some of us are born with a predisposition to being heavier or having medical problems such as high cholesterol or diabetes. However, lifestyle choices and environment also have a lot to do with your health. By environment, I'm talking about the day-to-day world in which we live; our jobs, relationships, kids, travel, and other factors that make healthy living a real challenge.

All the technological advances of the twenty-first century that were supposed to make your life easier have instead made life far more complicated and stressful. Compared to prior generations, we seem to have less and less time each day to take care of ourselves. And, that's how I found myself standing in front of the mirror facing the unpleasant reality that I had let myself slip into an unhealthy lifestyle.

I spent that week in Florida doing a lot of soul searching. I thought a great deal about health and longevity. I've always enjoyed writing, so my first instinct was to write down my thoughts. It was during that week that I created the outline for what would change my approach to patient care and would eventually become this book. Ideas flew through my mind as I started to see the connections between pieces of information that I had learned in my medical training and in medical practice. I started to understand the big picture of how wellness truly works in both the short and long-term.

A week later, I left Grandma Emma's Florida condo and flew back to Boston. I was eager to get back to my office and start sharing my enthusiasm and insights with my patients. I didn't quite know how to implement all of this, but I could sense it was starting to come together.

One of the first patients I saw that week was Victor, one of the most engaging and likeable people I've ever met. However, his overflowing enthusiasm and zest for life contrasted sharply with his extremely poor medical condition. He suffered from severe complications related to his long-standing type 2 diabetes including heart disease and recurrent skin infections in his legs. He was on an enormous list of prescriptions. Despite all of the medications, his medical problems still weren't adequately controlled because of his poor lifestyle.

Even though we discussed this at each office visit, Victor ate all the wrong foods in extremely large portions and lived a nearly completely sedentary life. Over the prior three years, we had many lengthy conversations about his high risk of having a stroke, heart attack, or even sudden death. Despite understanding all of this, Victor still hadn't changed his lifestyle. Victor's health was declining and we had reached the end of the line in terms of what traditional medicine could offer him. As I prepared myself to have the same conversation with Victor for the umpteenth time, I thought that there must be more that I could do to help him turn things around.

There I was in the exam room with Victor when, instead of again telling him what he needed to change, I decided to try something new. I asked, "Victor, what can I do to help you with this?" Victor didn't respond for about ten seconds. The silence seemed to last for an eternity. When he finally spoke, he said something that has stuck with me to this day. "Doc, I know what to do. I've read every diet book there is." Then he placed his hands around his belly and said "There's more to this than just knowing what to do. Please help me figure this out."

Victor then looked at me with defeat in his eyes and continued, "I want to be healthier, Doc. I just don't know how to do it. I don't know where to start, but if you tell me how to do it, I'll try. I'll give it everything I've got."

Basically, Victor asked me for an instruction manual for implementing a healthy lifestyle, much like the one that I had been working on since my Florida trip. I realized that Victor—and many of my other patients—needed something beyond being told to eat right and exercise. They needed a lifestyle plan that could be individualized and tailored to their needs, and that would provide both the information and practical advice for how to incorporate the plan into their daily lives.

That night, I took the outline I had written in Florida and expanded it to include every habit that I believed could help Victor and other patients like him. I challenged myself to create a comprehensive list of the habits that contribute to healthy living and longevity. As I constructed this list, I included habits that involved nutrition, exercise, sleep, and stress management. I also included habits from arenas that doctors don't normally address such as relationships, parenting, driving, and even spirituality. Most importantly, I made sure that each of these habits was backed by sound science and high quality published studies.

I continued to work on this for several months until I had created a patient handout that included the fifty most important, scientifically-validated lifestyle habits needed for good health. Each of the habits focused on tools and strategies for both short-term and long-term success. At the office, I was still seeing patients with the same problems such as diabetes, heart disease, and cancer, but now I was beginning to find ways to combine the medical care that I had learned at Johns Hopkins and Yale (mostly medications and procedures) with practical strategies for a healthy lifestyle.

This handout quickly became an integral part of my medical practice. During office visits with my patients, I discussed important lifestyle topics such as nutrition, exercise, sleep, and stress. With each patient visit, I tried to identify one or two lifestyle changes that would be most beneficial. I made sure that this was a collaborative effort so that these were habits that I felt were important and that the patient was interested in and committed to trying. At the end of each office visit, I wrote these habits on a prescription just like I would when I prescribed a medication. This lifestyle prescription became my patients' "homework" until the next appointment.

In Victor's case, he struggled with a sedentary lifestyle, so his first habit was to go for a five minute walk each morning. My goal was to make recommendations based on what was achievable and beneficial to the health of each patient.

In the beginning, I wasn't sure how this approach would be received by my patients. Would they be interested in my new expanded approach to health? Would they be willing to try some of the tools that I was recommending? The answer was a resounding yes! My patients actually started to change their habits—and improve their health—based on their homework from their visits with me.

Many of my patients started to take ownership of their health as they saw that they could make a true difference in their well-being. Patients shared the lifestyle handout with their friends and family members. Sometimes I would receive a phone call from a complete stranger to let me know that they had been given a copy of the handout by one of my patients and that it had changed their life.

In conjunction with appropriate medications and procedures, these habits helped my patients take better care of themselves. They achieved measurable improvements with diseases such as diabetes, cancer, heart disease, and autoimmune diseases. In addition to improving their chronic medical conditions, my patients also experienced tremendous success in losing weight.

I was thrilled this new approach was helping so many people. Patients like Victor, who had struggled with their weight for years, began to find the success that had eluded them for decades. In Victor's case, he lost approximately fifty pounds in the first year and then lost another fifty pounds the following year. His weight loss was the result of making slow, steady changes in his lifestyle habits. Victor looked and felt like a new person and his health was measurably improved in all areas. It was deeply gratifying to see him, and so many of my other patients, finally find the tools that he needed for long-term success.

While seeing such impressive results with my patients, I continued to add tools and strategies to the handout. I listened to my patients to learn what worked for them. I read dozens and dozens of journal articles each week searching for new and innovative strategies to add to the handout. I must have written several hundred drafts of that handout as I was determined to help my patients as much as possible.

Over time, I realized that the habits listed on the lifestyle handout represented timeless health principles that have always—and likely will always—support optimal health and longevity. Health is determined by a combination of genetics and environment: nature and nurture. In addition, there's a third component to the equation which creates the bridge between nature and nurture. That bridge is our habits. Our habits affect how our genetics are expressed in the environment in which we live.

In this book, you'll read success stories of how my patients have used these habits to improve their health and vitality. Some have lost impressive amounts of weight and are now in the best shape of their lives. Some have had incredible recoveries from autoimmune diseases, cancers, and heart disease. They've accomplished this by consistently practicing the principles contained in this book to find optimal physical, mental, emotional, and spiritual health.

The Wellness Code is not a diet book, but rather a way of life that leads to greater health and happiness. A common "side effect" of making these healthy changes to your habits is that you may be able to lose those nagging pounds that have been hanging around for all those years. No matter how many times you have tried to lose weight and improve your health, there's still hope that you can succeed. That's the hope that *The Wellness Code* offers.

I've been teaching this way of life to my patients, medical students, and colleagues for many years and I'm so thrilled that *The Wellness Code* is now available in book form. This book is intended to be as practical and implementable as possible—sort of like a good friend passing on some important information to you. My hope is that you will find yourself returning to this book as you seek your path to health and longevity by practicing these habits day by day, month by month, and year by year. I also hope that you will be inspired to pass on this information to others. One of the most effective ways to reinforce a habit is to teach it to someone else. Nothing makes me happier than seeing this information passed forward to someone else who may be in need.

We lost Grandma Emma in 2008, and there isn't a day that goes by that I don't miss her. I look back fondly on that 1998 trip to Florida and that conversation with Grandma Emma. That was my Jerry Maguire moment; the moment that changed my career and my life. Will this be your moment?

CHAPTER 2:

Why The Wellness Code Works and Diets Don't

The first step on your way to living *The Wellness Code* is to understand why diets don't work and why *The Wellness Code* works to achieve long term success in achieving an optimal weight, longevity, health, and happiness. Published research over the last several decades has consistently shown that standard diets are rarely successful for long-term weight loss. These studies have shown that only about 5-10% of dieters reach and maintain their goal weight after one year. This statistic is even more disappointing when considering that only about 3% of dieters have maintained their goal weight after three years. How about after five years? Sadly, less than 1% of dieters successfully maintain their weight loss after five years.

These medical studies have also shown that the majority of dieters end up heavier and less healthy after trying to follow a diet. Study after study has shown that diets are very unlikely to help people successfully lose weight or improve health. Once you accept that diets are not the answer, you can move forward and look for true solutions that work. The goal of this section is to explore the many reasons why diets don't work and why the tools and strategies of *The Wellness Code* work.

Small Changes vs. Big Changes

Most of us have made New Year's Resolutions to eat healthier and to exercise regularly. Despite the best of intentions—and sometimes the purchase of a costly gym membership—the majority of people are back in their old, unhealthy habits before March rolls around. Why is it so difficult to change habits?

The reality is that the adult brain is not designed to make drastic changes. While children are able to learn new skills almost effortlessly, adults are hard-wired to implement all the information and skills learned in childhood. Think about how easily children learn a new language or instrument. Human brains are like sponges during childhood but brain connections become generally cemented and fixed into place as you get older and it becomes difficult to learn complicated new systems.

The adult mind is wired to maintain the connections that formed earlier in life rather than to create complex new connections. This is one of the reasons that it's difficult to adopt a new diet or a new exercise program as an adult.

Now that you've heard the bad news, let me tell you the good news. The adult brain is able to make small adjustments quite easily. In fact, your mind craves small changes. That's why you love the latest smartphone, that new song, that compelling new TV show, or that new pair of shoes. A mature mind resists adopting new systems but welcomes small, manageable changes. Unfortunately, diets tend to ignore this simple truth.

Think of the wiring behind your TV or stereo system. It's simple to reconnect one or two wires. However, rewiring an entire sound system is much more complicated and difficult. Similarly, adults are usually successful at making one or two small changes at a time instead of trying to unplug their entire way of life and rewire their entire lifestyle in one fell swoop.

Allergy doctors take advantage of this concept when administering allergy shots. Let's say someone has an allergic reaction to cats, but still wants to keep their beloved pet. Their allergist may choose to prescribe immunotherapy, also known as allergy shots. The way this works is that a tiny speck of cat dander is injected into the skin of the patient. It's such a small amount that the person is unlikely to react to it. Each time the patient returns, a slightly higher dose is injected. Assuming that the patient doesn't have a reaction, the patient receives slightly higher doses of cat dander over time and this incremental process goes on for months or sometimes longer. The doses are increased so slowly that the body eventually comes to accept the cat dander as a welcome part of life and no longer reacts to it. The result is that the person can now be around cats without having an allergic reaction.

Well, that's how lifestyle change works. We accept small changes without much difficulty but reject more substantial changes. When small changes are made, the mind and the body accepts and welcomes the change as a member of the "family" and life moves forward embracing the new reality.

Stop looking for a completely new framework for life. Instead, follow *The Wellness Code* and keep your current framework while gradually changing your lifestyle over time. You will still strive to improve your lifestyle, but will do so in a way that is easy to implement and maintain over time.

Information Isn't Enough

Another reason that diets don't work is that most conventional diets simply provide information about what to eat and what to avoid. Similarly, most exercise and stress management programs focus on communicating information rather than strategies to adopt these habits for long-term success.

The Wellness Code provides the information about what you should do and also the strategies for how to implement these tools to transform your life. For a program to actually work for the long-term, it must go beyond simply providing basic health information. Most of my patients know exactly how to practice a healthy lifestyle, but struggle to implement what they know on a regular basis. My patients usually tell me that they already know what to eat when we discuss which foods to eat at each meal. When we work together to design an exercise routine, I again get that knowing look. Thus, it's clear that people need more than just information on what to do.

For example, if you're having trouble sleeping, you need to know more than just the recommended amount of sleep you should have each night. Identifying the need for more sleep is just the first step. You also need to know the specific steps you should take to increase the quantity and quality of your sleep. In this book, I will review both the "what to do" and the "how to do it" tools and strategies necessary to implement a healthy lifestyle into your daily life. *The Wellness Code* is all about helping you learn practical strategies to implement the changes you want to make in your life.

Tunnel Vision

Another reason why conventional diets fail is that they provide nutritional advice with tunnel vision—in complete isolation from other lifestyle factors. For example, one diet may instruct you to change one aspect of how you eat, such as limiting certain carbohydrates, without considering the impact of your other habits such as exercise, sleep, and stress. Practicing a healthy lifestyle needs to involve all aspects of your life—from eating to exercising to sleeping to your relationships to your spiritual practice. The hard truth is that we are doomed to failure if the focus is solely on nutrition. Nutrition is often a reflection of how a person's life is going. During times of stress or unhappiness, we often turn to comfort food and most diets ignore all of the other factors that affect how we eat.

Diets also typically try to find a gimmick to distinguish themselves. For example, one book tells you to eat more whole grains. Another book instructs you to avoid whole grains and focus on lean proteins. Another book claims that fruits and vegetables are the key to a long life. A different book tells you that the key is to combine your foods in certain ratios for optimal health.

These gimmicky programs rarely lead to a successful lifelong healthy lifestyle. A healthy lifestyle that supports wellness is an interdependent process where nutrition, exercise, sleep, stress, spirituality, personal relationships, work relationships, community relationships, and many other factors work together to promote health and longevity. All of these factors impact one another in either a positive or negative way. Life does not operate in a vacuum. True wellness comes from moving past the "diet" mentality and embracing a more comprehensive mindset. Start thinking of life as an interdependent world where each action leads to another action and so on and so on. The goal is to think of your lifestyle as a code or a way of life where you gradually shift your habits in a healthier direction.

Stages of Change

Whether you realize it or not, each time you change a habit, you progress through three major stages of change before the habit stays with you for life. Whether you want to stop biting your nails or want to start exercising, you will pass through three essential stages in order for that habit to become a part of your identity.

These stages of change are not addressed by most conventional diets or lifestyle programs. Understanding the stages of change is important to implement changes that will stay with you for life rather than those that come and go. For any program to work, you must consider the stages of change for each habit. One of the hallmarks of successful, permanent change is that the person has moved through the stages of change in the correct order.

Think about a habit you have changed at some point in your past, perhaps stopping smoking or beginning an exercise program. It may seem that you made that change all at once. In fact, you may remember the exact moment when you decided to throw out that last pack of cigarettes or you may remember the day you began to train for a marathon. Even though the final decision to change a habit may happen in a moment, the process leading up to that point usually occurs over an extended period of time. This time period involves a series of stages on your way to making that final decision to say "Yes!"

To delve a bit deeper into this, let's discuss the three major stages of change. Each of these stages includes smaller, more subtle levels, but the most important point to understand is that you must go through three major stages of change to have a habit evolve from where it is today to where you'd like it to be tomorrow.

1. Stage One: The Backstory

As screenwriters and novelists know well, the first stage of change is called the backstory. Most novels and movies begin with the protagonist living life in a certain consistent way. This lead character may be unhappy or happy, but life is stable, predictable, fully integrated and ordered. For example, you may be living a sedentary life in stage one of the change process. You wake up and go to work each morning, spend most of your day sitting at a desk, and then drive home each night. You may want to live a more active lifestyle or you may not have thought very much about becoming more active. Regardless of how you feel about being sedentary, you are in stage one so this habit is fully integrated into your current way of life and is unlikely to change without some effort or external stimulus. Stage one reflects the reality of what brought you to your present life.

2. Stage Two: The Shift

Stage two begins when something triggers a thought in your mind that things could be different. If this were a movie, something would happen to shake up your life and make things begin to change. In this hypothetical example, something triggers you to start thinking about becoming more active. Perhaps your spouse starts to exercise regularly or a friend joins a gym or you notice that your belt is getting awfully tight. Whatever the stimulus, something happens to you and you start to think that there's another way of life. You start to think a bit about exercise. You read some articles and talk to friends and family about it. You download a few exercise apps and start reading some blogs online. The idea starts to build some momentum in your mind and you start thinking about how you might fit exercise into your schedule. The shift has begun.

Initially, the journey to change doesn't involve giving up your prior way of life. While still holding on to your old way of life, you contemplate and then take baby steps towards becoming more active. Perhaps you buy a bicycle or stop by a gym to check it out. Maybe you start taking a walk after dinner or purchase a smart watch and start monitoring your daily steps. Slowly but surely, you start to practice what you have been contemplating.

During this stage, you begin to gravitate towards the new way of life and slowly start to move away from your old way of life. During this journey, you will encounter some high points where you feel great and also some low points where you feel lousy. However, you will gain motivation as you start to see what your new way of life will be like. You gain confidence that you can do this—that you can integrate this new habit into your life.

When you reach this point, you make the internal commitment that you're not going back to your old way of life. You cross the infamous point of no return as you have too much momentum to go back to your sedentary way of life. You've seen the new way of life and you're going for it. You have joined a gym or started working out at home. Perhaps you've purchased exercise equipment, such as an elliptical trainer, and now you're using it regularly. Your new exercise habit is becoming integrated into your daily life, but there's still one more obstacle to conquer which happens in stage three.

3. Stage Three: The New Life

Finally, you must win one last battle to be sure the new habit is fully integrated into your life. In terms of exercise, that final test usually happens when the excitement wears off and life gets busy at work or at home. It's at this point you will know if your new habit will stick. Will you push on and clear this last hurdle to make the habit a part of who you are? Or will you abandon the habit and retreat back to your stage one life?

In most movies, stage three is where the final confrontation happens. This is where the hero (that's you!) must prevail in a confrontation with the antagonist. In movies, the antagonist tends to be another person, place, or thing. In terms of habit change, the antagonist is usually within yourself—specifically inside your mind. How badly do you really want this new way of life? How badly do you want to give up your old way of life? Will you be all right without your old way of life? Are you afraid of what others will think? Are you afraid of how this new habit will affect other parts of your life? As you take this last step in the journey, the insecurities and questions in your mind will rise to the surface and make their last stand. This is where you need to stand strong and push forward and win this last battle.

When you arrive at the end of stage three, the habit is now fully integrated into your life. In this example, exercise has become a part of who you are. Exercise is now a fully integrated part of your routine just like showering and sleeping. Being active has become a part of your identity.

The final part of stage three is maintenance where you work to maintain this new habit as part of your life. With the exercise example, you now plan your schedule and your routine knowing exercise is a given. It's no longer optional; it's become an essential part of your life today and for the rest of your life.

Each time you successfully adopt a new habit, you go through all three stages of change. However, your starting point for each habit may be different. For one habit, you might start in stage one while you might start in stage two for another habit. As an example, you may be in stage one for eating a healthy breakfast, while you may be early in stage two for meditation.

Every lifestyle habit is at a different point in the stages of change and this needs to be factored into how you approach your habits. This is another place where conventional diets and lifestyle programs steer you wrong. These programs tend to assume that you are equally ready to change each of your habits as soon as you learn the program. The reality is that you're not. We'll review this in much more detail when we discuss the four column monthly process for habit change.

For now, the important point is that your habits are not all equally ready to be changed at a given time. Just as movies portray how a character progresses through a journey, it's helpful to think of each habit as being on its own journey. Thus, the path to wellness isn't just one journey, but rather many interdependent journeys. Now that we've explored why conventional diets don't work, let's begin to discuss *The Wellness Code* and learn why it works and where it fits into a comprehensive healthcare program.

One You vs. Two You's

One key to understanding *The Wellness Code* is the concept of the "One You" vs. the "Two You's."

When you learn a completely new program—such as a diet or an exercise program—a dichotomy is created in your mind. Two realities now exist in your mind, which I call the "Two You's." First, there's what I call the "Real You," which is the way you've been living your life up until now, including the sum total of all of your current habits. In your mind, this "Real You" represents your self-identity including all of your habits. You may or may not like this version of you, but you've grown accustomed to it and have accepted this as who you are.

One day, a new diet comes along and tells you that you don't need to be this old version of you any longer. The new diet says you can be a different person: you can be the "New You." In your mind there are now two versions of you: the "Real You" and the "New You." As you adopt this new diet, you try convincing yourself that you are no longer the old version of you. You begin to genuinely believe that you are now this new version of yourself. You start to think that you have become the "New You" and that the old version of you, the "Real You," is in the past and gone for good.

However, the old version of you isn't completely gone. It may be forgotten, but it's still there. In your mind, you're living life as the "New You," but the "Real You" still exists in the background. This creates a situation where you have the option of going back to your old way of life. You are outwardly living a new life, but deep down you feel like you're temporarily trying out a new lifestyle and know that reverting to your old way of life is an option. You're sort of like Clark Kent living an alternative life as Superman. You can be Superman for a while and follow this new program, but at some point you'll need to go back to your old life as Clark Kent.

For a given period of time, people can create a "New You" by following a set program. With discipline and focus, you can do things in the new way for a while, perhaps even a long time. However, this almost always turns out to be a temporary solution. The reason for this is that, in the back of your mind, you still view the "Real You" as your default program. Thus, when discipline inevitably wears thin and your focus fades, the tendency is to revert back to the comfortable "Real You." Your old habits find their way back into your life and the new way of life becomes a distant memory.

What's the answer? The key is not to have "Two You's." Don't look for a "New You," but rather maintain the "Real You" while gradually shifting your habits in the right direction. For most of us, it's a mistake to seek out a completely new way of life. Rather than adopting a program that involves changing everything about your life at once, instead tweak your lifestyle a little bit at a time—step by step, brick by brick, habit by habit. When you adjust your habits one at a time and gradually improve your habits and your health, you're much more likely to succeed in the long-term.

The secret of *The Wellness Code* is that you adopt one habit at a time, so there's no old version of yourself to which to return. There is no "New You." There is only one you: the "Real You." With *The Wellness Code*, instead of creating a new persona, you gradually shift yourself towards wellness. Because you make small, simple changes, there is no program to abandon. Over time, your lifestyle slowly grows in ways that have major benefits for your health.

For example, in childhood, your parents likely instilled in you the habit of brushing your teeth each morning and before bed. By adulthood, this habit is second nature. Brushing your teeth is simply a part of who you are. This is the optimal way to change a habit over time. One of the secrets to healthy living is to slowly adjust your lifestyle over time so there is no default program to which you can return. It's always the "Real You," getting healthier and happier over time.

Start thinking about each of your lifestyle habits and which stages of change each is in. As we progress through this program, you will adopt small manageable changes in your habits. This process works for long-term success as these small, simple changes become a part of the "Real You"—the same person, just healthier.

The Four-Legged Stool of Wellness

Before exploring *The Wellness Code* any further, let's take a look at the big picture and see where this fits into a comprehensive healthcare plan. To do that, I'll need to talk about some furniture: the four-legged stool of wellness.

I love metaphors, especially ones that clarify seemingly complex concepts. The four-legged stool is one of my favorite metaphors and I review this with patients because it helps to explain the four "legs" that affect your health.

Picture a four-legged stool where the stool represents your overall health and each of the legs represents a major component necessary for wellness. When the stool is intact, you can sit on it comfortably. However, when one of the legs weakens and breaks, the stool collapses and sends you falling to the floor. The stool can only support you when all four legs are intact and strong.

Each leg of this stool represents an essential factor for longevity, health and happiness. To have optimal wellness, you need all four legs of the stool to stay strong. Some people focus on only one or two legs of the stool and they believe that is sufficient to be healthy. However, just as with a physical stool, all four legs must be strong and intact or the entire stool can topple over. You need four strong legs to keep your metaphorical stool intact. The legs don't need to be perfect, but they need to be functional, intact, and strong enough to keep your stool upright. Let's review this in detail to better understand The Wellness Stool.

The Wellness Stool:
A Framework for Comprehensive Health

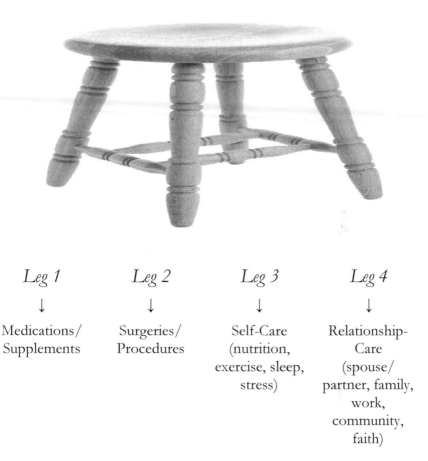

Leg 1	*Leg 2*	*Leg 3*	*Leg 4*
↓	↓	↓	↓
Medications/ Supplements	Surgeries/ Procedures	Self-Care (nutrition, exercise, sleep, stress)	Relationship-Care (spouse/ partner, family, work, community, faith)

You may have noticed that the first two legs have something in common: they represent the main categories of healthcare related to "Western medicine." These two legs are largely dependent on your doctor or healthcare practitioner helping you find the right combination of medications, supplements, screening tests, and procedures, as well as calling in a surgeon when necessary. The first and second legs, or the "Western medicine" legs, are critical for maintaining optimal health. I call these two legs *The Medical Code* and it is extremely important to work with a healthcare provider who is skilled in these two legs of the stool.

The first leg represents medications and supplements. This is what first comes to mind when you think of what doctors and other health practitioners usually prescribe. For a wide variety of health issues including infections, heart disease, and many other problems, the first leg of the stool can be essential to optimal health.

The second leg represents surgeries and procedures such as colonoscopies, hip replacements, blood tests, EKG's, x-rays, knee replacements, and many other surgeries and procedures. These have revolutionized health care and have contributed to the increase in life expectancy and quality of life that we enjoy today.

The focus of this book, though, is on the third and the fourth legs of the stool, which is what I call *The Wellness Code*. The third leg is the "self-care" leg and it encompasses all aspects of taking care of yourself: nutrition, exercise, sleep, stress management, and many other lifestyle elements. This is the leg where you have the most control over how you're doing. Unfortunately, some people don't do as well as possible with the third leg. They may eat too many high-calorie, high-fat, and highly processed foods. They may not exercise consistently. They may not get sufficient sleep. They may feel overwhelmed by stress. When people don't take good care of themselves, medical problems become more common. Strengthening the third leg of the stool is critical to maintaining and restoring optimal wellness.

I refer to the fourth leg of the stool as the "relationship-care" leg. This is the leg that has to do with how you care for all your relationships including your family, work, community, spiritual, and intimate relationships. If you experience a difficult situation—a job loss, a divorce, or the loss of a loved one—your health can be affected in all sorts of detrimental ways. Support from your friends, family, and community can help keep your wellness stool balanced and upright.

Medications and procedures are an important part of a healthcare regimen, but they represent only half of the stool. Practicing good self-care and having good relationships are also important components of a well-rounded, comprehensive healthcare program. By carefully examining your wellness stool, you can see how each leg can affect the strength of the other legs. An example of this is when a relationship stress occurs—perhaps a situation with a boss at work or in one's marriage or with a child. When this happens, many people start making poor food choices, sleeping fewer hours, or exercising less consistently. Thus, a weakness in one leg (in this case, the fourth leg) leads to a breakdown in another leg (in this case, the third leg). A breakdown in these legs of the stool can put you at increased risk of a medical problem such as an asthma attack, an infection, or even something more serious like a heart attack—any of which could necessitate a trip to the doctor's office or emergency room. At that point, you then have to rely on the first two legs (medication and surgeries) to pull you through the problem and help get you back on your feet again. However, in many of these situations, the problem could have been avoided in the first place with stronger third and fourth legs.

Keep all four legs of your stool in mind when you meet with your healthcare provider. Each component is vital to optimal health and longevity. A constructive doctor-patient relationship is a partnership in which the doctor and patient work in a collaborative manner to optimize all four legs. Before your appointments with your doctor, make a list of topics that you want to discuss. During your office visits, review which procedures may be of benefit to you, such as screening tests and ensure that your medications and supplements are optimized. Work with your healthcare provider to improve your nutrition, exercise, sleep, and stress levels.

The four-legged stool is the "big picture" of how to live a life of optimal health and longevity. Optimize all four legs and you've done all you can do to keep your stool healthy and upright—to maintain optimal health. Allow one or more of the legs to weaken and your health may weaken over time. Next, let's discuss the keys to putting *The Wellness Code* into practice in your life.

CHAPTER 3:

The Wellness Mindset

Picking up this book is a good indicator you are ready to make some positive changes. In the last chapter, I discussed the concept of the four-legged stool and how *The Wellness Code* fits into your comprehensive healthcare plan. Before going further, it's a good idea to take stock of how you approach your health and your habits by discussing the keys to being ready to improve your lifestyle. There are seven character traits which are vitally important to successfully implement *The Wellness Code*.

1. Personal Responsibility
2. Prioritization
3. Self-Discipline
4. Realism
5. Do The Right Thing
6. Self-Respect
7. Perseverance

As you read through the habits in this book, please keep these character traits in mind. Try to find areas in which you are already exhibiting these traits—those are likely to be the areas in which you are poised to make further improvements in your life. Also, look for other areas in your life where you might be able to apply these traits.

Character Trait 1: Personal Responsibility

Personal responsibility is essential for taking control of your life. This means that you don't place the blame for your failures—or the credit for your successes—on someone or something else. You are the captain of the ship of your life. You take responsibility for what happens: good or bad.

Most of us have heard the joke about two children playing in their room and one says to the other: "Mom better come in and get us up pretty soon or else we'll be late for school." This epitomizes how some people aren't proactive in taking charge of their lives and instead wait for someone else to take the lead. Ultimately, you are responsible for your own destiny. Don't wait for someone else, whether it's a spouse, office manager, or a friend, to tell you what to do. Evaluate your life and take responsibility for making changes when changes are needed. The choices you make have a profound effect on the outcome of your life. Effective life change is only possible when you take the lead in your own life.

Character Trait 2: Prioritization

In order to make meaningful changes in your life, you must decide what is important to you. One person might want to improve relationships with friends and family, while another might have nutritional and exercise goals. These are all worthwhile areas for self-improvement. However, before you choose a habit to improve, it is essential to first take inventory of your life and identify the areas that are important to you. Write down your to-do list of life goals—basically your bucket list for life. What happens if you never prioritize the items on that to-do list? Unless you consciously put those items first, it might turn out that you are prioritizing goals that don't add meaningful value to your life. Before you begin implementing any of the habits in this book, first write down what is important for you to accomplish in your life.

For example, when I began changing my life after that fateful conversation with Grandma Emma, this is what my non-professional bucket list looked like:

1. Get married
2. Have children
3. Run a marathon
4. Eat healthy foods
5. Get sufficient sleep

Writing down my life goals helped me realize that my lifestyle at the time wasn't conducive to achieving any of these goals and this inspired me to make some necessary changes.

What's on your bucket list? If you aren't sure where to begin, create your list while you read this book. As you come to a habit, decide if the area addressed by that habit deserves a spot on your priority list. This will help ensure that you spend time focused on habits that reflect your values and life goals.

Character Trait 3: Self-Discipline

How many successful people have to be nagged in order to do their work? Not many. Regardless of the arena in which the person has succeeded—business owner, musician, attorney, executive, stay-at-home parent—generally these are all people who are self-motivated and self-driven. They live their personal and professional lives in a proactive mode. They take responsibility for what needs to be done and then do it. Accomplishing this requires self-discipline: having the internal strength to stay focused on the job at hand. You can take personal responsibility and have priorities in life but you will only accomplish success if you have the self-discipline to do the necessary work to practice the habits that we'll be discussing in this book. Self-discipline is critical to long-term success.

One of the most important skills necessary for self-discipline is the ability to delay gratification. By this I mean having the ability to forgo what you want right now for satisfaction down the road. To give you a personal example, I enjoy listening to entire albums from my favorite music artists. Although the industry is moving away from selling albums and focusing instead on downloadable individual songs, I still enjoy the experience of listening to an entire album straight through.

It's particularly exciting for me when one of my favorite musicians releases a new album. In the "old days," it was a simple process of purchasing the album and playing the music. Nowadays, artists release one or more songs from an album in advance of the release date. This presents a challenge for me. Do I listen to these songs as they're released or do I wait a few months for the complete album so I can listen from start to finish? I usually choose the latter, but it takes tremendous self-discipline to not listen to the individual songs when they become available. I really want to hear them, but I know that doing so will detract from my ultimate enjoyment of listening to the entire album from start to finish. These sorts of situations arise all the time where you have a choice of instant vs. delayed gratification. Think about situations in your life where challenges like this may arise. When these situations come up, use them as opportunities to practice delayed gratification and strengthen your self-discipline. The more you practice, the stronger this skill gets, and the more successfully you will be able to succeed in your pursuit of optimal wellness.

Character Trait 4: Realism

In order to improve your health and find optimal wellness, you have to have an honest understanding of the reality of your life. Some people don't see their world as it really is but instead as they wish it were. For example, there are people suffering from extreme obesity who never look at their body in a mirror and never step on a scale. By carrying a mental picture of themselves of how they looked fifty or a hundred pounds ago, they can avoid having to acknowledge the reality of their weight gain. One reason why it's difficult to convince some overweight people to begin a healthy living program is that they haven't fully internalized the reality of their situation.

In order to decide what you'd like to change about your health and your life, you have to first have a realistic picture of your starting point. You know the saying: "If it's not broken, don't fix it?" If you don't believe something in your life is broken, you won't be motivated to change it no matter what other people are telling you. Thus, it is important to internalize a realistic picture of your life so you can move forward into a healthier future.

Character Trait 5: Do The Right Thing

In all likelihood, you probably like to think of yourself as an independent thinker—someone who doesn't just believe what others are saying or do what others are doing. However, each of us is influenced by our environment more than we realize.

Back in college, I took a class in social psychology where we learned about the psychology of how people act in groups and how they respond to their social network including friends, family, and colleagues. In classic studies, researchers simulated someone being injured to see if bystanders would intervene to help when they see others (actors) ignoring the situation. Unfortunately, when people saw the actors showing no signs of concern, the majority of people ignored the cries of the person who appeared to be injured. It was a sad testimony of how people are influenced by how others.

In the past, the main behavioral influence was mostly your group of friends, family members, work colleagues or religious group members. Thus, these were people you regularly saw as part of day-to-day life. However, now there's 24-hour access to the Internet and social media platforms such as Facebook, Snapchat, Instagram, Vine, LinkedIn, Twitter, etc. There are so many more external influences today than ever before and the Internet makes it easier for strangers to influence you. As a result, it is more important than ever to be careful about the influences that surround you and to be sure to draw your own conclusions about life. Of course, you should pay attention to the opinions of your friends, family members, colleagues, and those in your community, but ultimately you need to listen to your own moral code and act accordingly.

Many of the health problems we face today stem from people not making good sound rational choices. Thus, thinking for yourself and doing the right thing is crucial to your health and longevity. It is a key component to wellness. Listen to those you trust and whose experience you trust, but ultimately draw your own conclusions and act accordingly. Sometimes it takes bravery to follow your own moral compass instead of just following the crowd.

If you're sure to draw your own conclusions, you will be the one who intervenes to help someone in need. You will be the one to get up in the morning and exercise when others aren't. You will be the one to order the healthy meal when everyone else is getting the cheeseburger and fries. You will be the one who doesn't smoke that cigarette when others might be. You will be the one who doesn't gossip behind a friend's back when others are. Think for yourself. Listen to the experts. Listen to your friends. Listen to your family. Listen to those whom you respect. Take in all the information and then do the right thing.

Make it a practice to consciously evaluate situations and ensure that you aren't being overly influenced by other people. Think about some specific situations—food choices, gossiping, exercising—and make sure that you are thinking for yourself and making decisions that are in keeping with your values.

Character Trait 6: Self-Respect

It's unlikely is it that you will prioritize taking care of your health if you don't respect and care for yourself. Each person has inherent worth and it's so important that you internalize this truth. You must first value yourself in order to have a positive relationship with your family, your spouse or partner, your friends, and your community.

It's not realistic to expect other people to treat you well when you don't believe that you have tremendous value. In addition, people who respect themselves are better able to evaluate situations and make good life choices. People who value themselves are able to find situations and make decisions that add to their quality of life. Those with self-respect are also more likely to have the confidence to address the reality of their lives and to be able to determine what changes would enhance their lives.

Character Trait 7: Perseverance

What distinguishes successful entrepreneurs from people who have great ideas but never seem to actually turn their ideas into reality? Generally, it is the tendency to finish what they start and to refuse to quit when things get difficult.

Few things in life come without some degree of hard work and persevering though challenges. This holds true in both the business and personal realms. Most successful business owners can share stories of how they got through the lean years and survived the bad times. Most long-married couples and parents can share their experience of months and years where relationships caused more pain than pleasure and how much hard work it took to turn that relationship around. The common thread among successful people who turn adversity and challenge into a positive is that those people just never give up.

They take personal responsibility, prioritize what's important, apply consistent self-discipline, see life as it really is, do the right things, care about themselves, and persevere through tough times. These seven character traits are the "secret recipe" for success in practicing the art of healthy living. Please keep these traits in mind as I discuss each of the fifty habits of *The Wellness Code* as these are so important to the process of building healthy habits into your life. Next, let's discuss the habit-building process with a focus on the three steps needed to build long-lasting healthy habits.

CHAPTER 4:

The Three Steps to Habit Building

With the seven character traits to implementing *The Wellness Code* in place, the next question is: how do you shift towards a healthy, sustainable lifestyle while still living your demanding life? As I previously mentioned, you make this shift by gradually integrating healthy habits into your life in a way that is sustainable. In *The Wellness Code*, you will learn the fifty most important habits for living a life of optimal health, longevity, and lasting happiness. In this chapter, you will learn the practical strategies for incorporating these habits into your existing lifestyle. It is essential that you understand and internalize the skills presented in this chapter before you begin to practice the habits of *The Wellness Code*.

The practical steps necessary to change a habit and make the change last for a lifetime can be narrowed down to three steps:

1. Understand the habit
2. Practice the habit
3. Integrate the habit

This process of understanding, practicing, and integrating is at the core of each of the fifty habits that make up *The Wellness Code*. If there is a "formula" to transforming your life with *The Wellness Code*, this is it.

To develop expertise, whether in playing a musical instrument, driving a car, or learning a profession, you have to first understand the necessary skills. For example, if you want to become a talented piano player, you find an instructor to teach you how to play the piano with great proficiency. Without this musical education, all the practice in the world won't get you to Carnegie Hall.

Once you've attained the basic knowledge and understanding, the next step to achieve success is to practice, practice, and practice. You know this to be true in sports and in learning other skills—but somehow few people have accepted the need to learn and practice healthy habits over and over again for them to stick. Just as in other areas, you need to learn the skills required to be healthy such as making good food choices, exercising regularly, sleeping well, and controlling stress. This is much more than someone just handing you a schedule or a meal plan. You have to learn the right principles and then practice them over and over and over again.

After you understand the new habit and practice it repeatedly, you move on to the third step which is integration. In this step, the habit becomes a part of your fabric—an integrated part of your existence. You live these principles every day until they become a part of you, not simply a program that you're following. As previously discussed, you don't want to create a "New You," but instead slowly but steadily adjust your habits until they become a part of who you are. By thinking in these terms, there is no old you to which you can revert. There is only one you and that person is practicing and integrating new habits over time. The lack of integration of healthy habits is why most attempts at healthy living fail. Please read this sentence again because it may be the most important sentence in the book.

The lack of integration of healthy habits is why most healthy living programs fail.

You know what you're supposed to do. You may even know how to do it. You may even have a plan in place to get it done. However, for a habit to become fully integrated into your life, the habit needs to become a part of your routine just like showering, brushing your teeth, eating, or perhaps watching football on Sunday.

Practice these new habits day in and day out so that these principles become an integral part of your identity and won't be abandoned later. It's essential that these habits become a part of your routine so giving up the habit is no longer an option. Daily, consistent, sustained practice eventually leads to integration as the habit becomes fully incorporated into your life. The keys to strengthening and reinforcing the third leg of the stool are practice and integration.

This is important because it's easy to give up on a new habit when things get busy. During times of stress, you give up the things that aren't ingrained in your being. When life gets too hectic, it's easy to skip your exercise program or pick up unhealthy takeout food instead of preparing healthy meals. Generally, you give up the habits that haven't become integrated into your routine.

However, no matter how crazy life gets, somehow you always remember to shower and brush your teeth. When you are short on time, why do you continue to practice these habits on a consistent basis? The answer is that these habits have become integrated into your daily routine. Think about it: what do you give up when things get busy? What do you continue to practice consistently? The key to this entire process—and thus the key to a healthy lifestyle—is to find a way to integrate healthy habits into your schedule, your routine and your identity.

One of the most important tools to foster integration is automation which means doing something without conscious thought. Automation is an extremely powerful tool for creating consistent habits that last for the long-term. Once you've decided which habit you'd like to practice, find ways to make that habit an automatic part of your routine. Don't leave the habit to chance with the hope that you'll find the energy and motivation to practice it. Make the habit something that you do without thinking. Our goal is to find ways for you to practice healthy habits without having to think about them on a regular basis.

For example, let's say that you've decided to eat steel cut oatmeal with blueberries each morning. How can you create an environment so that a healthy breakfast is automated for you? One strategy is to make a huge portion of oatmeal on weekends and freeze it in single serving containers for later use. Each morning, you can quickly heat up a single serving and a delicious, nutritious breakfast is ready to go.

Automation may sound boring and repetitive, but it actually frees you up to spend your precious time and attention on more important parts of life. Rather than thinking about what you'll make for breakfast, you can stay engaged in what's most important to you each morning. Your attention and your creativity can be where they belong: focused on the people in your life and the projects that are important to you. Automation is a remarkable strategy that helps integrate habits into your life in a meaningful way.

Another key component of integration is to make the habit as specific as possible. By this I mean that the habit should be individualized and specific to each person. Sometimes people approach a habit in general terms and that can be a recipe for failure. For example, let's say you decide to practice habit 17, which is to practice aerobic exercise. You're not likely to have long-term success if you simply have a general goal to exercise. If an exercise goal isn't specific, it means that you will have to spend time each week deciding how often you should exercise and what exercise you should do. On the other hand, if you make a specific plan that you will exercise on your elliptical trainer for thirty minutes before work each morning, you are more likely to be successful.

In summary, these three steps—understand the habit, practice the habit, and integrate the habit—are the building blocks to successfully implementing healthy habits to create a foundation of optimal health and longevity. These three steps will be very important as you continue your journey through *The Wellness Code*. Now that I've explained the three steps to building a healthy habit, let's review the seven strategies that form the framework for successfully living *The Wellness Code*.

CHAPTER 5:

The Seven Tools for Living The Wellness Code

We've discussed the seven character traits necessary to live *The Wellness Code* and we've discussed how to use the three-step process to integrate healthy habits into your life. Next, let's discuss how *The Wellness Code* works in the real world. Over the years, I've developed tools and strategies to help my patients approach this process in a way that maximizes the likelihood of success. These seven basic strategies for success will help you to practice *The Wellness Code* on a daily basis.

1. The Four Column Process

The four column process provides the framework of how to bring *The Wellness Code* to life. As you read through and learn the habits, you will notice that some habits seem fairly easy to implement while others seem much more challenging. This is a highly personal process as the same habit may be easy for some people while challenging for others. The key to this process is to take note of your experience. Which habits seem easy for you? Which ones present challenges? This process will help you decide which habits to begin practicing in your life.

Before you begin reading the habits section of *The Wellness Code*, take out a blank piece of paper and divide it into four columns as illustrated below. As you read this book, use this paper to create a handwritten plan for implementing the habits. I recommend performing this process by hand as studies have shown that learning is optimized by writing things down rather than typing them into a computer, tablet, or smartphone. However, if you prefer to create your list through digital means, that can be helpful as well.

After you finish reading each habit in this book, list the habit in one of four columns as follows:

- **Column One:** includes the habits that you're already practicing consistently and are already integrated into your routine.

- **Column Two:** includes the habits that you're ready to practice at the current time.

- **Column Three:** includes the habits that you want to practice but aren't yet ready to attempt.

- **Column Four:** includes the habits that, for whatever reason, you don't want to practice.

Example of The Four Column Process

Column 1	Column 2	Column 3	Column 4
Consistent Habits	**Ready To Try**	**Maybe**	**Not Interested**
Habit 1 – correct # calories	Habit 3 – downsize eating	Habit 11 – clean calories	Habit 21 – plan calendar
Habit 2 – correct type calories	Habit 4 – ADAPT	Habit 12 – weigh yourself	Habit 23 – safe driving
Habit 13 – automate eating	Habit 5 – eat before eating	Habit 14 – slow down	Habit 32 – read a book
Habit 15 – avoid alcohol	Habit 6 – easy healthy food	Habit 16 – physical activity	Habit 38 – community
Habit 19 – stretching	Habit 7 – eat breakfast	Habit 17 – aerobic activity	Habit 42 – let go of pain
Habit 25 – do not smoke	Habit 8 – read the label	Habit 18 – weight training	
Habit 27 – allergy-proof	Habit 9 – healthy restaurant	Habit 20 – meditate	
Habit 28 – find joy	Habit 10 – prepare own food	Habit 29 – practice hobbies	
Habit 33 – volunteer weekly	Habit 22 – dental hygiene	Habit 30 – simplify your life	
Habit 35 – love spouse/partner	Habit 24 - anticipation	Habit 34 – love yourself	
Habit 36 – love your children	Habit 26 – sleep well	Habit 37 – love friends/family	
Habit 40 – live your values	Habit 31 – take a day to relax	Habit 46 – visualize	
Habit 43 – live within means	Habit 39 – find mentors	Habit 49 – forgiveness	
Habit 44 – integrity	Habit 41 – practice faith		
Habit 47 – practice gratitude	Habit 45 – leave a legacy		
Habit 48 – power of music			
Habit 50 – practice mindfulness			

Sorting the habits into these columns will help you see what changes are most important to you and which changes you're most ready to tackle. I recommend using a pencil rather than a pen as you will be shifting habits to different columns over time. In addition, I suggest you keep this list visually prominent to you if possible—perhaps on your refrigerator door, at your desk, on your night stand, as the screen saver on your phone, or on your bathroom mirror. The key here is to find a way that you will be prompted to review your list on a consistent basis.

Once you have the habits sorted into the four columns, review the list with a focus on columns two and three. First, review the second column, which are the habits that you're ready to practice on a consistent basis. Make note of what you'll need to implement each of them. For example, let's say you want to incorporate the habit of eating a healthy breakfast each day. What would you need to do to make this a reality? Do you need to go to the grocery store to stock your kitchen with some new breakfast items? As you review column two, make a separate list of everything you need to make each habit a reality.

Sometimes as you do this, you realize that items that you initially placed in column two truly belong in column three (or vice versa). Once you finish reviewing the habits in column two, move on to column three which are the habits that you're not quite ready to practice yet. For each item, list reasons why you're not ready to practice it consistently. Is it a time issue? Is it a family issue? Is it a motivation issue? Is it a scheduling issue? List all the reasons for each habit and think about these reasons and whether any of them can be overcome.

Finally, take a look at the fourth column which lists the habits that you don't want to adopt. For the fourth column, list the reasons why you don't want to change each habit. Many times the habits listed in the fourth column provide insight into your priorities.

This four column exercise is helpful in understanding which habits are realistic for you to address. I recommend that you perform the four column process on the first of every month and adjust your four columns as discussed above.

Over time, you'll find that some habits shift to the left towards column one. Some habits will move quickly while others take more time. Don't get frustrated if things don't progress as quickly as you'd like. Change takes time. *The Wellness Code* is not a quick-fix program. Rather, it is a long-term plan that helps you to slowly move forward to a healthier place.

2. Order From The Menu

Now that you've created your columns (or updated them if you are returning to this exercise for your first of the month column review), the next step to create your plan for the month. I call this process "ordering from the menu." To do that, review the first two columns as if reviewing a menu at a restaurant. Take a look at your four column "menu" and start by reviewing the first column, which contains the habits that are already a part of your life. Double check to ensure that all of these habits still belong in column one and haven't regressed into column two. Then review the habits in column two and pick two habits that will be your habits for the month. I generally don't recommend working on more than two habits at once. It's usually best to pick the habits that are the easiest to incorporate into your daily life. Just as it's easier to pick apples from the bottom branches of a tree, these are the habits that are most "ripe" and ready to be incorporated into your life. "Low hanging fruit" are the habits that are easiest to integrate into your life at the current time. That being said, you should also prioritize the habits that are most important for your circumstances.

On the other hand, if a habit appears too difficult at this time, put it on the back burner. You can consider it again in the future. Don't try to force yourself to work on a habit before you are ready, as that is a setup for failure. Focus on the habits that are ripe and pick those.

Once you've selected your two habits for the month, spend a little time to figure out how you will practice those habits on a consistent basis and also think about how you will integrate them into your life. Remember that practice and integration are the keys. How will you get these two habits to be a part of your life? How will you make these habits a part of who you are?

You adopt these habits by making small changes so they become a part of your routine. The changes you make shouldn't seem external to you. If you feel like you are twisting yourself into a completely different person to follow a program, then stop and re-evaluate. Remember the "Two You's?" The goal isn't to create a "New You" but rather to make small adjustments in who you are so the changes are likely to stick for the long-term.

Next, spend the month working to integrate these two habits into your life. Your goal for the month is simply to do the best you can with the goal that these two habits will become a part of your routine by the end of the month. Don't try to be perfect. As you progress through the month, stay engaged with how things are going. What's working? What's not working? If necessary, make adjustments in your routine. Be honest with yourself and maintain communication with those who are close to you. Enlist support for encouragement and accountability whenever possible.

When the month ends, review how you did with the two habits of the month. If you succeeded with integrating these two habits, congratulations! It's wonderful if both habits are now part of your routine, but don't stress if they aren't. If the two habits aren't yet a part of your routine, then remember that change takes time and doesn't always happen right away. For example, the average smoker tries to stop smoking seven times before finding long-term success. If you didn't do as well as you had hoped, brainstorm for ideas that may help you succeed with these habits in the future. If you think of changes you'll need to make to have success with these habits, do your best to make those changes.

Either way, start your next month by doing your monthly four column review. Review all the habits and move them between columns if any circumstances have changed. Think about each of the habits and make a fresh assessment of each one. As before, focus on the habits in column two and choose two new habits for the next month. You may choose to work on the same two habits as the prior month or you may want to start with two fresh habits. I usually counsel my patients to stay with the same two habits from the prior month if progress was being made. However, trust your instincts with this. Go with the habits that you feel ready to tackle given your current circumstances.

If you find that several months have gone by and you still seem to be struggling with a certain habit, then think seriously about whether this habit truly belongs in column two. Perhaps it really belongs in column three. Regardless of what you decide, be sure to choose two habits for each month and get started again.

Don't beat yourself up if adopting a given habit is more difficult than you think it should be. It's best to accept that you're going to struggle with some of these habits. As mentioned, focus on the habits that are most attainable to you. The great news is that as you grow and progress, habits that previously seemed impossible will likely become easier to achieve.

This process repeats monthly, so each month you get a new shot to make two habits a reality. As I've mentioned, this is a long-term process.

Stay upbeat and positive. Keep striving to improve your habits while at the same time embracing and accepting that no one is perfect.

3. The Unintended Consequences of Changing Your Habits

As you work on changing your habits, it's important to think through the unintended consequences that might occur as you exchange old habits for new ones. This is something that many people forget to consider as they work to optimize their lifestyle habits.

For example, if you decide to bring a healthy lunch to work each day instead of eating a high calorie meal from the cafeteria, you will need to think about how you can still maintain your lunchtime relationships despite this change. Perhaps you could bring your lunch and still join your colleagues in the break room or cafeteria. For many people, lunch meetings are an important part of the workday and it's essential to ensure that your healthy eating goal doesn't isolate you professionally. For lunch meetings at a restaurant, try to influence the choice of location so there is a healthy option for you to order. Other strategies are to have a big glass of water with lemon at meetings to help control your hunger, to eat your healthy lunch before these meetings, or to have some sugar-free gum during the meetings to help control your hunger. The key is to make a plan for how you can compensate for the inevitable collateral changes that result from shifting your habits.

Any modification to your habits inevitably results in changes in your life that may pose new challenges for you. Try to anticipate how things will play out and how you might be affected. Advance planning will increase the chances that you will be successful in sustaining your new healthier habits.

4. Remove Roadblocks

Another key to successfully change a habit is to consider potential roadblocks for your new habit and to come up with strategies to address these challenges.

Let's again use the example of bringing a healthy lunch to work each day. To make this work over the long term, you'll need a regular plan for your meals each week. Think about all the possible roadblocks that might get in the way. Do you have a strategy for purchasing these meals each week? Is there a refrigerator at work and, if so, is it large enough to stock a week's worth of meals or will you need to bring your lunch each day? Do you have a plan for beverages? Do you need to find a variety of lunch options or are you the type to enjoy the same meals over and over again? Can you partner with someone at work to ensure that you have lunch plans each day? Does your schedule allow for you to consistently eat lunch or do you need to block off your schedule for lunch each day?

For any habit you select, think through all potential roadblocks and then plan out ways to remove obstacles so you have the highest probability of success.

5. Announce The New Habit

Once you've chosen your two habits for the month, going public with your plans is a way to increase your likelihood for success. I know this may sound a little nerve-wracking, especially if you're not sure that you'll be successful, but telling others about your new habits is one of the most helpful actions you can take. When you publicly tell others about your plan to adopt new habits, you accomplish several important goals. First, you make yourself accountable. You are much more likely to persevere when others are aware of what you're doing. Second, it means that the topic is likely to come up occasionally in conversation, which provides a gentle reminder about your new habit. Third, there is the pass-it-forward concept. This means that if you tell someone that you're trying to exercise five times a week, you may motivate others to do the same.

In addition, one of the most powerful ways to cement a habit into your life is to teach it to others. Teaching something to others helps you gain true mastery over a subject and also increases the likelihood that you will stick to your new habit. Try teaching one of your habits to a friend, family member, or colleague. Teaching encourages you to look at information in new ways and serves to amplify and reinforce your learning process. Look for opportunities to announce your efforts to others: whether it be face-to-face or via social media platforms. However you decide to go public with your plans, this is an important step in successfully adopting your new habits and creating a support system to help you move forward.

6. Do It Now

Once you've chosen your habits and announced them to others, the next step is to just do it. Don't get bogged down in over-thinking or over-researching your new habits as this can become a form of procrastination. Generally, it's best to just jump in and do it now.

Sometimes planning and overanalyzing can be excuses to delay giving new habits a try. When you've settled on your two habits for the month and have the basics in place, announce it and then get started.

7. Linkage: An Important Tool for Successful Habit Change

One more tool that helps integrate a new habit into your routine is linkage. I first learned about linkage back in my early 30's when I decided that I wanted to run a marathon. The thought of finishing a marathon seemed like an amazing experience to check off my bucket list, but the reality of the long training runs was not appealing in the least. Since completing a marathon was something that I wanted to do, I came up with some strategies to make this happen. The most important strategy that I used was to link enjoyable activities to running. I decided to bring the joy of my favorite hobby—listening to music—to the not-so-fun long runs that were a part of my marathon training.

I created mix-tapes (of course now it would be called a playlist) of my favorite songs and listened to them while I ran on a treadmill. When one of my favorite artists released a new album, I waited to listen to it until I was running. Once I linked the two activities of music and running, I found myself enjoying running and actually looking forward to it. The sounds of my favorite bands and radio stations kept me excited about running. Music became my reward for running. Before long, I was on my way to running and completing a marathon. This was how I discovered the power of linkage.

Can linkage help you? Think about ways that you can link activities that you already enjoy with habits that you'd like to practice consistently. Some prefer audiobooks while others prefer music or a TV show. How can you make linkage work for you?

CHAPTER 6:

The Wellness Code

Now let's begin the exciting, fun part of this process which is to explore the fifty habits of *The Wellness Code*. It's a step-by-step path from where you are today to a healthier you—the same you as before but healthier and happier. The key to succeeding in this journey to wellness is to add habits in a slow, steady manner and to integrate these new habits into your life. *The Wellness Code* is comprised of fifty interdependent habits, each of which contributes to good health. As you learn about the fifty habits, begin the four column process by listing each of the habits in one of the four columns. Each month, you will work on two habits to help you reach your weight loss goals, achieve optimal health, and find lasting happiness.

Also, the discussions of each habit are intended to be basic introductions. They are not exhaustive or comprehensive in nature. The goal with each is to provide a summary of the basic principles and help steer you in the right direction as you integrate each habit into your life. For further exploration of each habit, I've provided hundreds of scientific references and recommended readings, which are listed at the end of the book. I've carefully chosen these books and research articles to ensure that they are consistent with the principles and practices of *The Wellness Code*. Please remember that, although knowledge is very important, it is the consistent practice and integration of each of these habits that is most important to long-term success.

In addition, throughout the book you'll be introduced to many patients who have benefited from the habits of *The Wellness Code*. The names and identifiable details of these patients have been changed in order to protect their identities. I hope you're excited to get started with this process. Let's start with habit 1.

Habit 1: Eat the Correct Number of Calories

Everyone knows that eating healthy foods is important, but figuring out how to actually accomplish this can be bewildering. We are constantly bombarded with conflicting information. One study supports the benefits of a low-fat diet. Another study supports the benefits of a low-carb diet. Another study supports the benefits of a high-protein diet. All of this information is intended to help, but the end result is just confusion.

Let's cut through all the nutritional trends and fads by focusing on the principles that are at the core of nutritional wellness. Health eating involves two components:

1. Eating the correct number of calories
2. Eating the correct types of calories

The first habit of *The Wellness Code* is to eat the right amount of food—specifically the correct number of calories. Most people don't know how many calories they should eat in a day. However, the balance between calories consumed and calories burned is the single most important determinant of whether you gain or lose weight. Sounds too simple to be true? A 2009 Harvard study placed patients on four different types of diets with varying amounts of carbohydrate, protein, and fat. These diets were meant to approximate the various popular "diets" on the market and the researchers followed these patients for two years. At the conclusion of the study, the Harvard researchers found that no matter which nutritional plan the patients followed, the one factor that best predicted weight change was calorie consumption.

The first habit in the healthy living process is to figure out how many calories you should consume and then to monitor your daily calorie consumption to ensure that you're achieving that goal. Your ideal caloric intake depends on many factors, including age, gender, height, weight, medical history, medications, and activity level. Before making any changes, be sure to meet with your personal physician to determine how many calories you should consume each day. Most people's target calorie consumption is somewhere between 1,400-2,400 calories per day.

Calorie tracking programs on smartphones, tablets, and computers can make keeping track of your calories easy. Popular apps and online programs include Lose It, My Fitness Pal, Calorie King, and Spark People—some of these programs are free or very low cost and most have databases that include common foods from both grocery stores and restaurants. These programs provide a reasonably accurate estimate of how many calories you should be eating each day based on the specifics of your situation and your weight loss goals. Another option is a wearable device from companies such as FitBit, Basis, Apple, Jawbone, Garmin, and Withings. The advantage of these devices is that they track both your caloric intake as well as how many calories you burn each day. These trackers can also track other habits such as sleep. All of these programs make it simpler to make smart food choices, whether you're eating at home or at a restaurant. They can be particularly helpful in picking restaurants as you can review menus before arriving. Moreover, these programs store lists of your favorite foods and beverages making it easy to re-enter the information once you've created these lists.

Research studies show that monitoring your calories doubles your chances of effectively losing weight and reaching your optimal weight. First, monitoring calories makes you accountable. When you're accountable, you're more likely to make good choices. Second, it makes you aware of a food's nutritional value. You are likely to improve the quality of your diet when you see the amount of calories, fat, sugar, and salt in what you're eating.

❖ ❖ ❖

In many cases when I recommend that a patient use an app to monitor nutrition, their first response is usually, "I don't have time to track what I'm eating." That's what my 43 year old patient Steven told me when we first discussed his weight. Despite considering himself a generally fit person, Steven's weight had slowly drifted up 30 pounds since college. Steven traveled a lot for work and was finding it more and more difficult to maintain a healthy weight.

I asked Steven if he would agree to use a fitness app to monitor everything he ate and drank for just one week. I told him that it would take about twenty minutes per day to document his food and beverage choices, but that this would be one of the most important habits for him to practice. Studies have consistently shown that monitoring calorie consumption doubles the chances of reaching and maintaining an optimal weight.

After a lengthy discussion, Steven agreed to try a food

tracking app for a week. At the end of the week, Steven called and told me he had learned more about nutrition in one week than he had learned in his entire life. He couldn't believe how many calories were in some of the foods that he was eating, and he was also amazed at how much fat and sugar were in some of his favorite nighttime snacks. Steven came back to see me six months later and had lost 24 pounds. At that point, he was using the app to monitor his food consumption on Wednesdays and Saturdays and this worked quite well to keep him on track. Steven had essentially the same schedule for most weekdays and an entirely different schedule for most weekend days, so monitoring his nutrition this way worked well for him. He told me that he had completely removed certain items from his diet and the weight seemed to peel right off of him. Small changes lead to big results.

◆ ◆ ◆

Remember to review your dietary plan and your daily calorie goals with your doctor or healthcare provider. You can also estimate your daily calorie goal with the apps and websites that I previously mentioned. Once you set your daily calorie target, monitor your consumption on a consistent basis to make sure you're consuming the optimal amount of calories.

I recommend starting by tracking everything you eat or drink for one week. Adjust your diet over time to keep your calorie consumption in line with your goals. Once you settle into a routine, track your food intake one weekday and one weekend day per week for maintenance.

If you need to lose weight, consume 100-200 fewer calories than you burn each day. Reducing your intake more than this may be tempting, but can lead to undue hunger and cravings and reduce your chances for success. If you are already at your goal weight, ensure that your calorie balance (calories in vs. calories out) is even.

Does it matter which calories you consume? Are all calories the same? Is a calorie of broccoli the same as a calorie of a cookie? The answers are in habit 2: eat the correct types of calories.

Habit 2: Eat the Correct Types of Calories

There is more to healthy eating than simply the net balance between calories in and calories out. Nutritionists are often divided into two camps when it comes to determining what constitutes healthy eating. Within the first camp are those who focus mainly on calories. The second camp of nutritionists focuses less on the number of calories and more on the nutritional value of each calorie. As in most areas of life, the truth lies somewhere in between. It is important to find a balance between consuming the correct number of calories (habit 1) and consuming the healthiest types of calories (habit 2).

In the previous habit, I discussed the importance of eating the correct number of calories each day. However, all calories are not created equal. Some calories are chock full of nutrients and promote good health while other calories are overly processed and are loaded with unhealthy sugars or fats. A small cookie may have the same number of calories as a cup of broccoli, but clearly the broccoli is a much more nutritious option.

In addition to consuming the correct number of calories each day, you also want to focus your food choices on calories that are "nutrient-dense." A convenient list of these foods can be found at the end of this section. The majority of your calories should be from these foods as they are loaded with healthy nutrients which nourish your cells and your health. These are the calories that promote health, longevity, and optimal wellness. Avoid "nutrient deficient" calories which have little nutritional value. Examples of "nutrient deficient" foods include cookies, pastries, breads, and highly processed foods.

Of course, when deciding what foods are appropriate for you, you should first consider your own unique situation. Any food to which you are allergic or sensitive should be avoided. Foods that elicit an allergic or sensitivity reaction contribute to inflammation and aging and are not healthy choices for you.

Nutrient-dense foods include an assortment of options such as spinach, broccoli, kale, tomatoes, avocados, apples, peaches, oatmeal, Greek yogurt, ocean-raised salmon, egg whites, legumes, almonds, walnuts, garlic, berries, and olive oil. These are just some examples of healthy calories and there are many other tasty, healthy options to consider.

You may have noticed several commonalities among each of the foods that I mentioned as being nutrient-dense. First, "good calories" are real food. They appear on your plate pretty much in the same form that they emerged from the Earth. A good rule to remember is that whenever food is processed, it loses nutritional value.

A good example of this is oatmeal. In the grocery store, you will find many different types of oatmeal, with the healthiest type being steel cut oatmeal that typically takes about thirty minutes to cook on the stove. Steel cut oatmeal means that the oats have not been processed, so what you see is what you get. The oat was cut into pieces instead of rolled flat during the manufacturing process so you get all the healthful qualities of the oat. Rolling the oats requires a steaming process that may remove some important nutrients.

You will also notice instant oatmeal where you simply add water to the oatmeal powder. This sort of oatmeal is a decent breakfast option, but most instant oatmeal has been highly processed. A good rule of thumb is try to purchase oatmeal with the fewest listed ingredients. In general, the fewer the ingredients and the more often the word "whole" is used, the more nutritious and less processed the product is. Start thinking of your food choices in these terms and try to choose the least processed, most nutrient-dense foods whenever possible.

Second, "good calories" tend to be colorful. UCLA's Dr. David Heber wrote a very useful book called *What Color Is Your Diet?* in which he discusses the health benefits of eating foods of a variety of colors such as reds, oranges, yellows, and greens. In general, the more colorful foods tend to be the foods richer in nutrients while the less colorful foods—the "white foods"—tend to be the more processed, less nutritious choices.

Third, "good calories" tend to be more filling. When you eat good calories, you're more likely to feel satisfied and be more in control of your portion sizes. One of the main reasons so many people gain weight is that their portion sizes are simply too large. Foods that have little nutritional value don't contribute to making you feel full so you are likely to eat large portions. However, simply eating a variety of nutritious, colorful foods makes it much easier to feel full and to keep portions under control. No matter how delicious, it is more difficult to overindulge in a salad than in cheesy lasagna.

As a part of the discussion about getting the optimal amount of nutritional value out of foods, I should also bring up the role of vitamins and supplements. Supplements are generally extremely popular, but take a secondary role in *The Wellness Code*. We've previously discussed the four-legged stool model of comprehensive care where the second leg of the stool includes supplements along with medications. Thus, supplements do have a role in the care of some patients, but let's explore this in more detail.

Vitamin A, vitamin E, vitamin C, and other vitamins, are extremely important to the functions of life. For your brain to work properly, you need to have sufficient vitamin levels in your bloodstream and internal organs. For your muscles and heart to work properly, you need sufficient vitamin levels. The same applies to your immune system. Many studies show that people who don't have sufficient levels of certain vitamins have a significantly greater risk of medical problems. Also, there are many studies showing that cells in a laboratory setting function better when certain vitamins are added to the cells.

However, remember that these studies are performed in a lab and are not clinical trials involving real people in real life conditions. It is very interesting that vitamins don't seem to be nearly as helpful when we look at high quality clinical trials. How can we reconcile the fact that adding vitamins appears to help in the laboratory, but not so much when tested in people?

It has always seemed odd to me that we would assume that just taking a vitamin by itself would provide the same health benefit as getting that vitamin from food. The reason is that life doesn't work in a vacuum, but in a complex, interdependent way.

For example, when you eat an orange, you get far more nutritional value than just vitamin C. The orange provides many other vitamins and cofactors necessary for the vitamin C to work properly in the human body. In addition to vitamin C, oranges contains vitamin A, thiamine (vitamin B1), riboflavin (vitamin B2), niacin (vitamin B3), pantothenic acid (vitamin B5), vitamin B6, folic acid (vitamin B9), choline, vitamin E, calcium, iron, magnesium, manganese, phosphorus, potassium zinc, lutein, and flavonoids. For the vitamin C to work properly and provide optimal nourishment to your body, it must be accompanied by the other vitamins, minerals, and naturally occurring cofactors that are found in an orange. This is why isolating and purifying one vitamin doesn't seem to work nearly as well as eating the foods that are rich in that vitamin. There are exceptions and circumstances where certain supplements are needed. However, vitamins and minerals should generally be obtained through food whenever possible.

The goal is to start thinking of life as an interdependent world where each action leads to another action, and another, and so on. Isolating individual elements ignores the reality of how life really works and the relationships that exist between each component of nutrition. As you focus your attention on eating foods with the most nutritional value, it is also essential to pay attention to how nutrition interacts with other elements of a healthy lifestyle such as exercise, sleep, stress, relationships, and so on.

The flip side to this is to understand which foods you should avoid. The general rule is to avoid processed, empty-calorie foods such as white rice, pasta, bread, preservative-rich prepackaged foods (cookies, pastries, and candy bars), and high-fat animal products (especially processed meats). If these foods dominate your diet, it becomes challenging to consume the optimal number of calories each day. Foods devoid of nutritional value do little to reduce cravings and can actually increase hunger and lead to overconsumption.

For instance, many people think that diet soda can help limit calorie consumption and be a part of a healthy weight loss program. However, it turns out that consuming diet soda actually increases your chances of gaining weight. How can that be? Diet soda speeds up your digestive system creating a sort of laxative effect which makes food move through your stomach more quickly. More rapid movement of food through your digestive tract means your stomach empties more quickly, leads to increased hunger, and makes it more likely that you'll eat too many calories.

One thing to keep in mind when you seek to eat the "good calories" is that beverages such as soda, juice, and alcohol can take up a huge portion of your daily caloric allowance without adding much in the way of nutritional value. When you stick with nutrient-dense foods, you're much more likely to keep your calorie consumption in line. These foods tend to be naturally low in calories, so you can eat more food and feel satiated. In addition, these foods provide a variety of important nutrients.

Sarah is a 27 year old executive assistant at a top movie studio in Los Angeles. She came to see me because she lacked energy and had gained about 35 pounds over the last couple of years. Sarah felt fatigued in the afternoons, especially after eating large meals heavy on carbohydrates, such as bread and pasta. She also mentioned that she was urinating more often and was more thirsty than usual.

Blood testing showed that Sarah was diabetic. Her diet rich in simple carbohydrates had triggered her genetic predisposition for diabetes. I explained to Sarah that her increased urination reflected her body's efforts to clear the excess sugar from her body. Her choice of empty carbohydrates such as bread and pasta raised her blood sugar and did not provide essential nutrients like phytonutrients and vitamins. Sarah asked me which supplements would provide those nutrients as she wanted to continue to eat the same foods and use supplements to fill in her nutritional gaps. I explained that studies have shown that the optimal way to get these important nutrients is by consuming foods that naturally contain them, rather than by taking supplements. Fruits and vegetables are examples of carbohydrates which are plentiful in healthful nutrients.

Sarah and I spent some time reviewing her food choices and finding foods to substitute for the bread, pasta, and sweet snacks she had been eating. I suggested alternative food choices and she said that she was excited at the idea that just a few dietary changes, along with medication, could help control her diabetes. Fortunately, when we rechecked her blood work three months later, her sugar levels had returned to normal. Sarah was excited to see such great results and to have been able to dramatically improve her health by making lifestyle changes along with a medication. Over the next year, Sarah did so well that we were able to discontinue her medication. Moreover, her sugars remained in the normal range with a healthy lifestyle program based on the habits of *The Wellness Code*.

❖ ❖ ❖

Try your best to choose nutrient-dense, colorful foods that are packed with antioxidant and anti-inflammatory properties. Replace "white foods" with foods such as fruits and vegetables, legumes, fish, and lean chicken. Get as much color as possible onto your plate. Aim to have a salad either with lunch or dinner. Make fruits and vegetables your snack foods of choice rather than processed options like candy, crackers, or chips. Have a bowl of oatmeal with some berries (such as blueberries, blackberries, and cranberries) each morning.

I've created a list of my favorite nutrient-dense foods which are listed in the accompanying chart.

Dr. Morris' Nutrient-Dense Foods

Apples	Artichoke	Arugula
Asparagus	Avocado	Beans
Beet greens	Blackberries	Blueberries
Broccoli	Brussel sprouts	Cabbage
Cauliflower	Chicory	Collard greens
Cranberries	Edamame	Egg white
Fish	Flax seeds	Grapes
Greek yogurt	Chicken	Kale
Legumes	Lentils	Mustard greens
Nuts	Oatmeal	Olive oil
Peppers	Pomegranate	Pumpkin
Quinoa	Radish	Raspberries
Sesame seeds	Spinach	Squash
Strawberries	Sweet potato	Swiss chard
Tofu	Tomato	Turkey
Turnip	Watercress	Zucchini

The CDC also has a list of foods that contains a high level of nutritional value and this list can be found in table 1 at the end of the book. Moreover, a list of the protein content of various foods can be found in table 2.

It's also important to make sure that you have the optimal mindset when it comes to making food and beverage choices. By this, I mean that you should make your choices based on what is most nutritious rather than what is most tasty. Many of us grew up making food choices based solely on taste. Comfort food is based on eating what you think would taste the best and make you feel a certain way. Sometimes you just feel like a cookie, a steak, or a slice of pizza. Of course, food should taste great, but taste shouldn't be the only basis on which you decide what to eat and drink. Your choices should instead focus on what is most nutritious for you. Making choices based on what is best for you is a major paradigm shift in the direction of wellness.

The next time you open the fridge, try not to focus only on what might taste better, but instead think about what might be best for you. That doesn't mean that you always reach for a kale salad, but be sure to keep your health in mind when making food choices as often as possible. You will find that this shift in your mindset will help you be successful over time.

Remember the two general principles for a healthy nutritional plan: eat the correct number of calories and also make these calories as nutritious as possible.

Habit 3: Downsize Your Eating Habits

In the first two habits of *The Wellness Code*, I reviewed the importance of eating the correct number of calories each day (habit 1) and making sure that your calories are as nutritious as possible (habit 2). However, there's more to healthy eating than just your daily calorie goal and a list of good and bad foods because environmental factors also influence food choices. Whether you realize it or not, what surrounds you influences how you feel and act. However, many are unaware of how much of an impact their environment has on them.

When asked, people usually say that they eat when hungry and stop eating when full. Most of us believe that our internal state determines how much we eat. However, in study after study, it turns out that environment has a huge impact on how much you eat. Much of this research has been done by Brian Wansink and is well-summarized in his classic book *Mindless Eating*.

One of Dr. Wansink's findings is that plate size has a tremendous impact on food consumption. In one study, reducing the diameter of the plate by just two inches reduced the number of calories people ate by about 22%. This means that you will generally eat less if you eat your meals on smaller plates. Try placing your dinner on a large plate and then transferring your food to a smaller plate and you'll see how different the meal looks. On the large plate, the meal looks like a relatively average sized portion. On the small plate, the meal looks quite large and much more satisfying.

In addition, it's simply easier to put more food on a larger plate, so portion sizes on a larger plate tend to be larger. When using a smaller plate, you need to make the conscious decision to fill up your plate again if you want to have a second portion. If that second portion is already on your plate, then you're likely to go ahead and eat it. On the other hand, you may skip that second portion if it involves going back to the kitchen to fill up your plate. Skipping that second plate can sometimes be the difference of 200 calories in a day. Remember that 200 fewer calories per day over the course of a year translates to about twenty fewer pounds on the scale.

It's not just the size of your plate that affects how much you eat. The size of utensils, serving containers, cereal boxes, and bowls all affect the quantity of food you eat. Reducing the size of these items can reduce caloric intake by upwards of 30-40%. The beauty of this habit is that it's passive. You don't have to even think about it. Simply substitute smaller utensils, smaller plates, and smaller serving containers and you'll immediately find that you have reduced your portion size.

Phil is a 48 year old executive who came to see me because he had gained ten pounds over the past six months. He told me that he had always been able to avoid gaining weight by making smart food choices. Phil was frustrated that he was gaining weight despite eating all of the "right" foods.

Phil provided me with his food diary from the past month and it looked like his choices were fairly sound. His diet was focused on fruits, vegetables, and lean protein choices like grilled fish and chicken. He avoided empty calories and most of his beverages were water. However, I noticed that his food diary didn't include portion sizes—it simply listed "grilled fish with asparagus" or "dinner salad without dressing."

When I asked Phil about portion size, he gave me a "deer in headlights" stare and told me he had never really thought about it. I asked Phil to use one of the apps on his phone to estimate how many calories he had eaten the previous day. I returned a few minutes later to find Phil sitting in shock after realizing that he had consumed 3,600 calories in one day. We determined that he had burned 2,600 calories during that day so he had eaten 1,000 calories more than he burned in just one day. Extrapolated over one week, this extra 7,000 calories would amount to a gain of about two pounds.

Phil realized that, although it was important for him to make good choices about the quality of his food, it was also important that he make good choices about the size of his portions.

Habit 4: The ADAPT Process

This habit will teach you how to actually accomplish your goal of consuming the correct number of calories for your situation. The way that I teach my patients to do this is by using a process that I call the ADAPT process. This process is so important that it's a separate habit in *The Wellness Code*. Let's review how this works.

Step 1 is "A" which is to "Assess" how many calories you're currently consuming. Whether using an app, an online tool, or a handwritten food journal, track all food and beverages you consume each day for a week. See habit 1 for details about how to practice this and try to accurately estimate your portion sizes. Be sure to include hidden sources of calories like ketchup, mayo, salad dressing, and beverages.

Spend the first week simply tracking your caloric intake. At this point, don't try to change what you are eating; simply document how many calories you consume each day. A full week's assessment usually provides the most complete picture of your diet.

Step 2 is "D" which is to "Downsize" your calorie consumption. Of course, to appropriately downsize your calories, you need to know how many calories you should be consuming in a day. If you haven't yet calculated your optimal daily caloric intake, please refer back to habit 1 for more information on how this works.

Once you've documented and reviewed what you've eaten for one week and have set your daily calorie goal, try to find easy ways to bring your calorie consumption into balance. Can you reduce portion sizes? Perhaps you can make simple food substitutions, such as having a salad instead of a sandwich. Perhaps you can drink unsweetened iced tea instead of juice. Find these simple swaps to downsize your caloric intake.

Step 3 is "A" which is to "Automate" your eating and Step 4 is "P" which is to "Plan" in advance. These steps—Automate and Plan—go together because they are so intertwined. Once you see how you could have done things differently, plan out how you can accomplish these changes going forward. You may have to go shopping and buy different foods and beverages. You may have to prepare more of your meals at home. Once you plan out what you will do, automate the process. Make healthy eating as simple possible so you don't have to think as much about your food choices. For example, bring a salad to work so you don't have to think about what you'll eat for lunch. Prepare food over the weekend so you have lunches and dinners ready for the upcoming week. The goal is to plan your meals in advance as much as possible and then to automate your meals so you will have healthy options readily available to you.

Step 5 is "T" which is to "Tell" others what you're doing. To do this, tell at least one person you are making changes in how you're eating. There's a significant power that comes with sharing what you're going to accomplish. It can be a friend or a family member or a co-worker or even a Facebook status update. Make sure that you feel comfortable communicating what you're doing, but try your best to find people with whom you can share your efforts.

Remember, ADAPT means to Assess your daily calorie consumption, Downsize your calories, Automate and Plan so you can achieve your goals, and finally Tell at least one other person what you're doing.

Following the ADAPT model can be life-altering and can make your goals attainable.

Habit 5: Eat Before You Eat

If you want to control portion sizes and make healthy choices at mealtimes, eat a healthy snack before each meal. A few years ago, researchers at Penn State University published a study where they asked participants to eat a small snack fifteen minutes before lunch. They were either given an apple, apple sauce, or apple juice. These pre-meal snacks were equivalent in calories, but had very different effects on the patients. Those who were given an apple consumed 187 fewer calories with their lunch than those who ate nothing before their meal. And here is the real kicker: this calorie savings included the calories from the apple. This benefit was not noted when participants were given apple sauce or apple juice.

Other studies have found similar findings. For example, one study found that those who consumed vegetable soup before a meal consume about 130 fewer calories with that meal, accounting for the calories from the soup.

In another study, participants who ate a large, low-calorie, healthy salad (about 3 cups) before lunch consumed about 10% fewer calories with the meal (salad calories included) than when they didn't have the pre-meal salad.

Studies from Scotland have shown that chewing gum prior to meals significantly reduces calories consumed during that meal. The effect is not as potent as the "apple effect," but still significant. In the Scottish studies, patients consumed on average about 50 fewer calories with each meal which translates to about a ten pound weight loss in one year if applied to lunch and dinner each day for a year.

Why are these measures so effective and so important? The act of chewing is a powerful appetite suppressant. Most people think the brain only senses that you're full when your stomach fills up with food. However, it's much more complex than that. When you chew, the nerve endings in your jaw muscles send signals to your brain letting you know that you're eating and your appetite drops. This is why even chewing gum reduces appetite.

Make it a habit to use the "apple effect" to your advantage. Chew on a piece of fruit or a small healthy salad before your biggest meal of the day. When an apple isn't available, try chewing some sugarless gum before a meal. The gum is especially valuable when traveling or going to a restaurant. Eating before you eat is a secret weapon as you try your best to keep your portion sizes and calorie consumption in line.

❖ ❖ ❖

Pam is a 38 year old attorney who takes several medications for high blood pressure, yet still struggles to control her blood pressure. Pam's stress level was also extremely high and was intensified by a recent promotion at work. During an office visit, she asked me if losing some weight might help control her blood pressure.

Pam had gained about fifteen pounds over the last five years. I told her that getting back to her ideal weight might help manage both her stress level and her blood pressure. We then reviewed her current lifestyle with a focus on her dietary choices. One thing that jumped out at me was that most of her calories were consumed at dinner. She typically ate a small healthy breakfast such as bowl of oatmeal with almonds and a small healthy lunch like a well-balanced salad with just a sprinkle of dressing. We calculated her calorie consumption from breakfast and lunch and it averaged out to be only about 750 calories.

In stark contrast to her breakfast and lunch, her food choices and calorie consumption in the evenings were generally unhealthy. Pam told me that she tends to be very tired and hungry when she arrives home from work and ends up snacking on chips because she doesn't have the energy to make a healthy dinner.

I suggested to Pam that she try making it a rule to have a small apple and an eight ounce glass of water as soon as she gets home each night. Just as eating an apple takes time, drinking water also takes time and both of these activities helps slow you down and allow times for your appetite to be reduced.

Two weeks later, Pam called and told me she was ecstatic with her success. She said eating this snack made her feel much more in control. It took the edge off her hunger and allowed her the time and energy to prepare a healthy dinner. Pam also reported that her total calorie consumption at dinner was significantly reduced. She was on her way to reaching her weight goal.

Habit 6: Make Healthy Food Convenient

When healthy food is convenient, you are much more likely to make healthy choices. Accordingly, habit 6 of *The Wellness Code* is to make it as easy as possible to make healthy food choices. The natural tendency is to choose foods that are in closest proximity to you. Have you ever been to a Super Bowl party with snacks such as cookies or chips on the table right in front of the TV while more healthy options remain in the kitchen? Do you overindulge in those snacks or do you head over to the next room to prepare a healthy snack? The main reason most people reach for the snacks on the table is convenience.

Cornell University researcher Brian Wansink illustrated this in his study measuring chocolate consumption in relationship to proximity. In an office setting, he first put a bowl of chocolates right on peoples' desks. He then moved the bowl of chocolates to a drawer inside the desks. Lastly, he put the bowl inside a cabinet across the room. What happened? You guessed it. Moving the chocolates from the top of the desk into a drawer reduced consumption by about 30%. Moving them from the desk to the cabinet across the room reduced how much people ate by about 50%.

We are all busy. Human nature is such that, when presented with several options, more often than not you tend to take the easier option. So if it's 8 p.m. and you're tired from a long day and you have the option of going to the gym or watching your favorite TV show, which will you choose? Some of the time you'll head off to the gym. Usually that happens when your focus and discipline are fully engaged. However, when you're tired and worn out from a long day, you may be more likely to grab some food and watch some television. This is why it's so important to make healthy food options as convenient as possible.

Years ago I saw an interview with former NFL head coach Bill Parcells. When asked for his secret to coaching success, he said that it was to put each player in a position where they had a high likelihood of succeeding.

If you know you have a sweet tooth and you are trying to cut your sugar intake, don't have cookies or cake around the house. If you know you like to overindulge in Chinese food, don't have leftover Chinese food in the fridge. If you know your healthy eating goals are getting sabotaged by your nightly habit of enjoying a cold beer, don't keep beer in the house. It's as simple as that.

It's far easier to make the decision to not purchase a certain food at the grocery store than it is to resist eating it every night. Keep pre-cut fruits and vegetables ready in the fridge for you to munch on at night. Have plenty of other healthy food options available at home or at work. When you make healthy food and beverage choices convenient, you greatly increase your chances for success.

If you want to have a salad each day for lunch, think of ways that you can make salad readily available. Prepare or purchase salads in advance and store them in the refrigerator so you have the salads ready to go each day for lunch. When lunchtime comes, all you need to do is head to the fridge and your healthy, delicious lunch is waiting for you. Put yourself in a position to succeed by applying these principles to all areas of your life. Bring lots of healthy meal and snack options to work or wherever else you spend significant time. Make healthy food options accessible to you at home, work, and when you travel. In addition, make unhealthy food options as inaccessible as possible. It's best to do so by keeping the unhealthy choices where they belong: in the grocery store.

◈ ◈ ◈

Dorothy is a 57 year old generally healthy patient who came to see me for a check-up. During her visit, she asked for advice about her overweight brother Ted, who struggles with diabetes and high blood pressure. When Dorothy recently visited Ted, she was shocked at all the snacks and processed foods in the house. Ted said that he wants to remove most of the unhealthy foods from the house as he doesn't have sufficient will-power to resist eating them. The problem is that Ted's wife Sandra enjoys eating snack foods and wants to keep them in the house. Sandra cannot understand why Ted can't just resist eating unhealthy foods.

For Ted, having these snacks in the house is sort of like asking a newly sober alcoholic to go out for happy hour and refrain from drinking. Dorothy asked for advice to help her brother. My suggestion was that he should remove these foods from the house. If that's not possible, I recommended that he should make these foods as inaccessible as possible. Literally put them on a high shelf or inside a box so that he won't see them and be tempted. Studies have shown that this simple measure can decrease the likelihood that the person will eat the unhealthy food.

A few weeks later, Dorothy called me to say that Ted had taken my advice to move the snacks to less accessible areas in their pantry and he was doing much better with his eating. This simple change had made such a positive change for Ted that Sandra was now considering removing some unhealthy foods from the house. This one small change had created momentum that was shifting their home environment in a healthier direction.

◆ ◆ ◆

Habit 7: Eat Breakfast

Your mother was right that breakfast is the most important meal of the day. In published studies, eating a healthy breakfast reduces calories eaten per day by about 100 calories, reduces cholesterol levels, and helps control blood sugar levels. It's a win-win. You get to eat and get healthier at the same time.

Why is breakfast so important? When you go long periods of time without eating, your body produces hormones that put you in "starvation mode." These hormones help conserve energy and place your body into a long-term savings mode that favors fat storage rather than fat metabolism. If you finish dinner at around 8 p.m. and don't eat again until lunch the following day; you've gone about 16 hours between meals, which puts your body into a "starvation" response. This state promotes weight gain—particularly fat accumulation around the mid-section. Fat in the mid-section is particularly detrimental in that it is associated with diabetes and atherosclerosis increasing the risk of heart attacks and strokes. It also contributes to inflammation which is linked to various types of cancers and autoimmune disease. This is why it's important to have a healthy breakfast each morning.

What is a healthy breakfast option? There are many great options including protein shakes, Greek yogurt, high fiber/low sugar cereals, oatmeal, fruit and nuts. Eggs have gotten a bad rap over the years, but can be a part of a healthy breakfast several times a week. Egg whites are a great protein source and also a good source of vitamins and important minerals. The egg yolk does contain some cholesterol but also contains some important nutrients as well.

When shopping for cereal, pick one that contains whole grains. Look at the first two ingredients listed on the box. The word "whole" should appear there to signify that the whole grain was used. A whole grain contains three different parts (bran, endosperm, and germ) each of which provides different important nutrients. When grains are refined (made less than whole), some valuable nutrients are lost in the manufacturing process. These lost nutrients may include fiber, protein, vitamins, minerals, or other important parts of a healthy diet.

A non-profit organization called The Whole Grains Council independently assesses cereal and oatmeal products and calculates how many whole grains are in each serving. Look for their gold label on product boxes. In general, it is ideal to consume at least 48 grams of whole grains per day.

Cold cereals have come a long way in the last twenty years and there are now many good options to consider. Look for The Whole Grains Council logo and find cereal with low calories, low saturated fat, high fiber, high protein, and good taste.

❖ ❖ ❖

James is a 49 year old marketing executive who wanted help losing weight. After some discussion, it was clear that lunch was his major challenge. His day typically includes a catered lunch with his clients or eating out. Both of these options tend to be high in calories and light on nutrition. Unfortunately, James doesn't have input into the catering choices or the restaurants where his meetings are held. James told me that he usually has a couple of cups of coffee with milk and sugar for breakfast. When lunch rolls around, he's extremely hungry and it finds challenging to limit his portion sizes. James also told me that his energy level drops by mid-afternoon, so he grabs another cup of coffee—often with a muffin or scone—so he can get through the rest of his day.

I recommended that James eat a healthy breakfast each morning, and we reviewed various options that fit his taste and schedule. We focused on ensuring adequate protein and fiber in his breakfast options to help maintain satiety through the morning. We also reviewed some filling, low-calorie, high-protein options to have as a late morning snack to further limit his hunger by lunch time. This way, James could head into his business lunches with his hunger under control and the ability to limit his portion sizes. These strategic measures helped James reach his weight loss goal over the following months.

❖ ❖ ❖

Eat a healthy breakfast each morning. If you're really cramped for time in the morning, consider quick options such as a prepackaged protein shake or a low-sugar protein bar along with a piece of fruit.

Habit 8: Read the Label

I've alluded to nutritional label reading in several prior habits, and this is the sole focus of habit 8. The trick is that you need to understand how to quickly read and assess food labels and then make your purchasing decisions based on this information. Food labels include a significant amount of vital information so you can easily figure out what's healthy, what's not, and what's somewhere in between. This makes it easier to make an informed decision when shopping at the grocery store so you can be sure to generally bring healthy options into your home. This is important because the chocolate ice cream calling your name is easier to resist one time at the grocery store rather than every time you walk past it in the kitchen.

It can be difficult at first to read those nutritional labels, but don't let them intimidate you. To help you make healthier choices, I'd like to share my 7 step crash course on nutrition label reading that you can use as you shop at your grocery store or online. Before you know it, you will soon have a healthy kitchen. When you're looking at a nutrition label at the store or online, go through the seven steps to determine if this is a product that you should consider purchasing.

◆ ◆ ◆

The 7 Step Crash Course on Reading Nutritional Labels and Choosing Healthy Foods

1. **Total calories per serving.** The first step is to look at calories and serving size. Make sure you are aware of the serving size as the listed calories usually—but not always—correspond to one serving. Remember your total daily caloric goal (habit 1) so evaluate each item to determine whether the number of calories fit into your plan. If yes, move on to the rest of the label. If not, put the item back on the shelf and look elsewhere.

2. **Saturated fat.** Daily saturated fat should be less than twenty grams. There is some wiggle room in this recommendation as it mostly pertains to animal-based

saturated fat rather than plant-based fats. In terms of fats, most people simply look at the total amount of fat per serving. Instead, I recommend choosing foods with healthy fats (monounsaturated fats, some polyunsaturated fats, and some plant-based saturated fats) and avoiding unhealthy fats (animal–based saturated fats and trans-fats).

3. **Trans-fat (should always be zero).** Total daily trans-fat intake should be as close to zero as possible. If an item has trans-fats, leave it at the grocery store.

4. **Fiber (should be greater than three grams per serving if possible).** Total daily fiber should be twenty-five to thirty grams. A 2011 study showed that those who consume the most fiber have a 22% lower risk of death, especially if the fiber comes from whole grains.

5. **Sugar (should be less than five grams per serving or as low as possible).** Total daily sugar should be less than thirty grams. Some companies disguise the amount of sugar by using terms such as "sugar alcohol" or "corn syrup." When calculating total sugar, include both simple sugar (listed as "sugar") as well as other sugars listed under other names because all of these sugars behave similarly in the human body.

6. **Protein (should be greater than three grams per serving if possible).**

7. **Sodium (should be as low as possible).** Daily sodium intake should be less than 2300 mg.

---------------------❖ ❖ ❖----------------------

If a food passes each of these seven steps, then it has earned a spot in your shopping cart and in your kitchen. If not, put it back on the shelf and keep shopping!

———————————◈ ◈ ◈———————————

Julia is a 36 year old stay-at-home mom who came to see me for a check-up. As we were discussing her health, Julia noticed that I keep empty food boxes—such as oatmeal, high fiber cold cereal, and a pre-packaged lunch—in my examination room. I explained that these boxes were there to teach patients how to read nutritional labels. We spent the next fifteen minutes reviewing the basics of nutritional label reading. We reviewed each line on the label and discussed how to interpret the information and make smart choices. Although Julia was clearly interested in learning about this, she confessed to me that she had never really looked at a food label prior to that day's office visit. After reviewing several labels, Julia told me that she was shocked at how much nutritional variation there is amongst foods and she now understood how important it is to read labels.

Although she came for just a routine visit, she left the office that day with information that would alter the way her family eats for years to come. Julia called me a few days later to let me know that she had found healthier alternatives for almost every product in her home. Without changing anyone's eating habits, Julia was able to shift her family to a healthier lifestyle just by reading nutrition labels.

———————————◈ ◈ ◈———————————

Go through your kitchen and read all the food labels in your house. You may be surprised how many unhealthy foods have snuck their way into your pantry and refrigerator. After you've identified them, do your best to remove the unhealthy foods from your home. If you are reluctant to waste food, consider donating unopened packages to your local food bank instead of eating your way through the unhealthy food in your pantry.

From now on, read food labels when you shop and make it a habit to use the information to purchase healthier products. You may not initially love the taste of each new food, but give them a chance. As time goes on, some foods may start to taste better as your taste buds adjust to healthier choices. Buy an assortment of healthy foods and see what appeals to you. Reading nutrition labels is a key to making healthy nutritional choices.

Habit 9: Guide to Healthy Restaurant Eating

Dining out is one of the biggest challenges to healthy eating. In general, restaurant meals are less nutritious than meals prepared at home. According to a recent survey, the average Americans eats about five meals a week at restaurants. Since eating out or bringing home takeout food has become a regular part of life, it is essential to find strategies to stay true to your healthy eating goals while dining out.

The main priority of restaurants is to provide delicious food and an enjoyable dining experience. While there certainly are restaurants that do a good job of combining nutritious food with great taste, it's a safe assumption that most restaurant food is less nutritious than you'd like it to be. Numerous studies have shown that you eat more calories, unhealthy fat grams, sugar, and sodium when you eat at restaurants.

In an ideal world, you would eat out less frequently and prepare most of your own meals. I encourage my patients to reduce their number of restaurant meals in half. I would prefer if you prepare all of your meals at home. However, for most people, it's not practical or realistic to do so. Thus, it is important to find ways to ensure that your restaurant or takeout food is as healthy as possible.

My eight strategies for healthy restaurant eating provide an excellent starting place to help you accomplish this.

1. **Pick the restaurant carefully**. Now that most people have smartphones or tablets, evaluating restaurants has never been so easy. There are countless apps and websites that review both the taste and the nutritional value of the food at restaurants. Many restaurants also have their menus online so you can see what's available while you sit in your office or your home. Some restaurants even make their nutritional content readily available for you to view so you can evaluate options before you arrive. Read the menus and see if there are healthy choices that appeal to you and fit within your nutritional goals. It's far easier to make healthy choices if you plan in advance to ensure that a restaurant has healthy options. Otherwise, you can easily find yourself sitting at the table with only unhealthy items from which to choose.

2. **Know what you will order before you get there.** Typically, people arrive at a restaurant hungry. When you're hungry, you are much less likely to make good choices. You can avoid this problem by having planned your entire order before you walk into the restaurant. By using one of the apps mentioned in habit 1 or the restaurant's website, you can easily calculate how many calories the meal contains to ensure that you're staying within your optimal goal.

3. **Eat before you eat.** Ensure that you're not starving when you sit down at the restaurant. If you're famished, you're much more likely to grab the bread or order a high calorie appetizer or beverage. Be in control and be only moderately hungry. Consider eating an apple or have a big glass of water before stepping into the restaurant in order to keep your hunger at bay (habit 5).

4. **No bread.** Many restaurants love to put a basket of bread on the table so patrons can munch on something before ordering. However, this can add up to a lot of extra calories—easily 300 or more calories before your food arrives. Do your best to resist. Better yet, tell the server that you don't want the bread and to keep it away from the table. Having snacked on a healthy option before you arrive at the restaurant, your hunger should be under control. If you're still famished, check the menu for something healthy to munch on such as a small salad or some vegetables. Hopefully you've read through the menu in advance of your arrival and you know what healthy items you can quickly order.

5. **Order in stages.** In America we usually order our entire meal—drinks, appetizer, entree all at once. However, that means you're ordering when you're hungry and more likely to over order and then overindulge. Ordering in stages ensures that the food you order reflects your state of hunger throughout your meal. If possible, skip the appetizer and try to start with something healthy like a small salad and then reassess your hunger level. You may find that you want to order a regular entrée but you may decide that you feel satisfied and prefer to order something smaller for your main meal. Don't consider ordering dessert until after finishing your meal. Your appetite may have been completely satisfied at that point. Again, don't feel pressured to order too much all at once. Stay in control and order each part of your meal after you've eaten the prior course and keep making assessments of where you are hunger-wise.

6. **Control your beverage intake.** Be careful not to consume too many calories from your beverage choices. Sometimes I'll meet with a patient who tells me that he's only eating 1600 calories a day and can't understand why he hasn't lost any weight. So I'll ask him to use an app to count his calories for 24 hours and it often turns out that he didn't include beverages in the 1600 calories. Obviously, many beverages have significant calories and these calories count. Everyone knows that alcohol can be high in calories, but also remember that juice and soda can have a lot of calories. Since some restaurants refill drinks as a courtesy, it is easy to lose track of how many calories you are drinking. Watch your beverage intake and do your best to minimize the calories from beverages, especially as some can be full of sugar and light in nutritional content.

7. **Share a dish.** Another strategy related to ordering is to share dishes when possible. If you're at a restaurant with a good friend or your spouse, think of ways to share dishes rather than each person ordering a separate appetizer and entrée. Can you share an appetizer or an entrée? Restaurant portion sizes these days can be large and some dishes can easily provide two, if not three, portions. Speak candidly with your server about the size of the dishes and see if sharing might work for you. Of course, this isn't an option at a business meal but, if possible, consider sharing dishes. It can be a nice way to cut down your portion size and, as a bonus, also save on the cost of the meal.

8. **Use small plates.** As explained in habit 3, studies show that using smaller plates, bowls and glasses can help control portion sizes. Restaurant plates can be enormous and using a larger plate encourages you to eat more food. One defense against this is to use smaller plates at restaurants. The easiest way to accomplish this is to use the entree plate as a serving plate. Ask for serving utensils and a small plate and serve the food onto the smaller plate, which makes it easier to eat smaller portions. Forcing yourself to take that moment to decide whether or not to take another serving can help to curtail the size of your portions. When eating from the main plate, it is easy to just keep eating until all the food is gone. However, by having to take another portion from a serving platter, you create a breakpoint in the meal. This slows you down and gives you opportunities to stop eating if your body indicates that you've had enough.

Victoria came to see me because her snoring was disrupting her husband's ability to sleep and was affecting her marriage. An overnight sleep study showed that she had obstructive sleep apnea which is a serious breathing issue that compromises both sleep and, potentially, overall health. After a thorough medical evaluation, we used a two-tiered treatment approach for Victoria.

First, Victoria agreed to use a prescription CPAP machine, a breathing apparatus that ensures sufficient oxygen flow during sleep and also reduces snoring.

Second, we identified that Victoria's weight gain of twenty-five pounds over the past seven years contributed to her snoring. A lifestyle evaluation made it clear that Victoria's habit of eating out for about ten to fifteen meals a week—including both meals eaten in restaurants and takeout meals—was a big reason for her weight gain. Some quick calculations determined that eating out was adding an extra 700 calories a day. I encouraged Victoria to reduce her dining out to no more than three to five total meals per week and to make healthier choices when eating out. Victoria said that reducing her restaurant eating wasn't realistic for her lifestyle, but she did agree to use my guide to healthy restaurant eating to make better choices. Over the next six months, Victoria lost twenty-five pounds and noticed a remarkable improvement in her energy level and her snoring.

At a follow-up visit, Victoria commented on how much more energetic she felt. I asked her to imagine wearing a 25-pound belt and how difficult that would make it to breathe and walk. And then I asked her to imagine taking off that 25-pound belt and how liberating and free it feels. Being twenty-five pounds overweight is like wearing a 25-pound belt around your waist all day long. Thinking in these terms makes it apparent why you feel more energetic when you get to your optimal weight. For Victoria, the simple change of making healthier choices at restaurants made a major difference for her and set up her on her way to long-term success.

◆ ◆ ◆

Try your best to follow the above steps to make healthy choices, even when dining out. Also, think about reducing how often you eat restaurant food, take-out food, and leftover meals from restaurant food.

Habit 10: Prepare Your Own Food

This habit of *The Wellness Code* is a follow-up to habit 9 where I discussed ways to eat healthier at restaurants. Restaurants are wonderful for special occasions, but try to prepare your meals at home as often as possible. When you cook your own food, you have more control over the ingredients so meals tend to be prepared in a healthier manner.

Because it is usually not practical to make a home-cooked meal at 6 p.m. every night, I recommend planning ahead. Make dinners in bulk and freeze them so you have healthy frozen dinners available whenever you need them. Buy a programmable slow cooker so you can come home to a hot, healthy meal after a long day at work—the slow cooker can also be used to heat up your homemade frozen dinners. Spend part of a Sunday afternoon preparing a variety of healthy salads so you have healthy, homemade, "fast food" available. Implementing these ideas can actually make it less time-consuming to eat home-cooked meals instead of stopping for takeout.

◈ ◈ ◈

Stuart is a 40 year old high school teacher who came in for a check-up and I was surprised to note that his blood pressure was mildly elevated. As his blood pressure had always been normal, I asked about recent lifestyle changes and Stuart shared that, since the recent birth of his first child, he's been bringing home takeout food for dinner quite often. In the past, Stuart and his wife cooked dinner together every night. I told Stuart that his elevated blood pressure was possibly related to the high sodium content in those meals. Stuart agreed to go back to preparing meals at home for one month to see how his blood pressure would respond. I told him that I would prescribe a medication for his blood pressure if his readings remained elevated. Thirty days later, Stuart returned and proudly told me that they hadn't eaten out for the entire month. Remarkably, his blood pressure had completely normalized in that time. Stuart was thrilled to have found success without the need for a prescription medication.

◈ ◈ ◈

Prepare most of your meals at home. It's not as hard as it sounds, and you may enjoy cooking more than you think. Make cooking a family activity. Try cooking your favorite dishes over the weekend and then storing them for home-cooked meals throughout the week. You can also cook and freeze meals so you have quick home-cooked meals available whenever you need them. Cooking can be fun, so make it joyful time.

Habit 11: Eat the Clean Calories

There's been a lot of debate in recent years about our food supply and changes in the foods and beverages that we consume. For example, some foods have been genetically modified while other foods have undergone other changes such as hybridization. In addition, many of us are concerned about the pesticide content in some of the fruits and vegetables in our grocery stores. Moreover, food additives such as colorings, artificial sweeteners, and preservatives have become more common.

The next time you're in the grocery store, read some of the labels on various foods and drinks and you will be amazed at the number of chemicals. In addition to the chemicals listed on food labels—typically on processed foods—there are also unlisted chemicals in some of the foods in the supermarket, especially in fruits and vegetables. I am asked all the time about consuming genetically modified food, food colorings, and preservatives.

There has been some concern that these changes in our foods may be related to various health problems such as the rise in allergies, autoimmune diseases, and even cancers. At this point in time, there is no conclusive evidence to say that there is a relationship between changes in the food supply and these health problems. However, I do recommend that you do your best to minimize your consumption of these chemicals and modified foods, especially if you suffer from inflammatory conditions such as allergies or an autoimmune condition like psoriasis, eczema, inflammatory bowel, disease or other similar problems. If you have one of those conditions, your body already suffers from increased inflammation, and it is important to avoid any unnecessary chemicals as they can exacerbate inflammation. Inflammation is at the root of many health problems, including the big three: cancer, vascular disease (namely heart attacks and strokes), and autoimmune diseases. One of the most important health goals is to reduce inflammation and avoid exposure to those things that contribute to inflammation. Thus, avoiding extraneous chemicals and foods that may trigger sensitivity reactions is a priority.

Obviously, you should stay away from things to which you are sensitive or allergic, whether that's dairy products, wheat, or oak trees. Moreover, many people who are sensitive to one type of food or part of the environment are also sensitive to other things. Thus, it's best for people with sensitivity issues to avoid consuming extraneous chemicals. Food colorings, such as yellow dye #5, are a particular problem for some allergy sufferers, especially those who are allergic to aspirin or anti-inflammatories such as ibuprofen or naproxen. In addition, some people are also sensitive to other types of food colorings and additives. This is of particular concern as there is some evidence that additives in the food supply may be a trigger for some autoimmune diseases like Hashimoto's thyroiditis, psoriasis, and eczema.

Two simple steps at the grocery store can help you avoid chemicals in your food and beverages.

1. Go organic for the dirty dozen fruits and vegetables. One of the benefits of buying organic is that, in theory, the product hasn't been exposed to pesticides. A conventionally-grown apple has likely been sprayed with pesticides (sometimes multiple types of pesticides) while an organic apple has not. Most of the pesticides in your diet come from fruits and vegetables and it turns out that fruits and vegetables aren't created equal when it comes to pesticide content. Some fruits and vegetables contain excessive levels of pesticides while others contain a negligible amount.

The easiest way to minimize pesticide exposure is to be sure to purchase organic versions of the fruits and vegetables that contain the most pesticides. This information is available from EWG (Environmental Working Group) on their website EWG.org. These are the "dirty dozen" fruits and vegetables that contain the most pesticides: apples, strawberries, celery, grapes, peaches, spinach, sweet bell peppers, cucumbers, nectarines, cherry tomatoes, potatoes, and imported snap peas. Buying organic versions of these twelve fruits and vegetables will provide a very significant reduction in your pesticide consumption.

The "Dirty Dozen" Fruits & Vegetables

Apples	Grapes	Cucumbers
Peaches	Celery	Cherry tomatoes
Nectarines	Spinach	Snap peas – imported
Strawberries	Sweet bell peppers	Potatoes

From EWG's 2015 analysis of pesticide residue testing data from the U.S. Department of Agriculture and Food and Drug Administration. EWG's 2015 Shopper's Guide to Pesticides in Produce™

EWG also provides a list of conventionally grown fruits and vegetables that contain the least amount of pesticides. These are the "clean fifteen" fruits and vegetables. Remember that some fruits and vegetables, such as watermelon, bananas and oranges, have a fairly impenetrable coating that helps insulate the food from the pesticides so buying organic is less important.

The "Clean Fifteen" Fruits & Vegetables

Avocados	Onions	Eggplant
Sweet corn	Asparagus	Grapefruit
Pineapple	Mangos	Cantaloupe
Cabbage	Papaya	Cauliflower
Sweet peas (frozen)	Kiwi	Sweet potatoes

From EWG's 2015 analysis of pesticide residue testing data from the U.S. Department of Agriculture and Food and Drug Administration. EWG's 2015 Shopper's Guide to Pesticides in Produce™

Thus, a good rule of thumb is to buy organic for the "dirty dozen" fruits and vegetables and those that have an edible outside layer and to buy conventional for the fruits and vegetables where you discard the outer layer of the food.

2. Avoid products with food colorings, food additives and preservatives when possible. Read food labels and choose the foods with the shortest ingredient list and the fewest chemicals. Avoid foods with a lot of words you don't recognize, especially if they have colors in their names with numbers. Some of these chemicals are preservatives whose role is to increase the shelf life of the product. A good line to remember is, "The longer the shelf life, the shorter will be your life." This doesn't mean that you can never eat anything with food coloring or food additives. It's just prudent to avoid these when possible, especially for people with allergies, autoimmune issues, vascular problems, or cancer.

Other steps to minimize your exposure to chemicals include avoiding fish with a high concentration of mercury and avoiding foods that have been treated with hormones. How strict each person should be depends on their circumstances. The message for this habit is to do your best to avoid exposure to unnecessary chemicals. Eating organic for the dirty dozen fruits and vegetables and making a conscious effort to avoid food colorings is a good first step. These measures move you toward the goal of focusing on real food that is whole and unprocessed. That means that you should focus on foods that look like they did when they came out of nature and avoid foods that are in boxes with long ingredient lists. As always, I recommend that you discuss your individual circumstances with your personal physician or healthcare professional to best determine what dietary changes are best for you.

◆ ◆ ◆

William is a 38 year old accountant who came to see me because his wife was concerned that he was experiencing allergic reactions that caused his upper lip to swell. William had learned to take allergy medication like Claritin or Zyrtec as soon as he noticed tingling in his upper lip as that signaled the start of the swelling. As the medication reduced the swelling and he was able to somewhat control this reaction, William hadn't previously seen a doctor about this.

It became clear that he was experiencing angioedema—an allergic reaction that manifests as swelling of certain body parts. Angioedema is generally caused by an allergic reaction to specific medications, foods, or beverages. William had stopped eating shellfish because he often experienced swelling after eating foods such as lobster and crab. However, he still had angioedema episodes, usually at night and especially within a few hours of bedtime.

He and I reviewed his routine and I quickly suspected that his toothpaste or mouthwash might be causing this problem. We checked and found out that both products contain a dye called yellow dye number 5 which is also known as tartrazine. This dye is a common food coloring and has been associated with allergic reactions such as angioedema and can be a particular concern in people who are allergic to shellfish or aspirin. I asked William to change his toothpaste and his mouthwash to products that don't contain any artificial colorings. I also prescribed a medication for William to use in case the angioedema affected his ability to swallow or breathe.

A few months later, William called and told me his episodes of angioedema had stopped. He said that he had found yellow dye number 5 in many other items that he was using—such as chewing gum and snack foods—and had stopped consuming all of those products. After so many years of dealing with this problem, William was finally angioedema-free.

◈ ◈ ◈

Habit 12: Weigh Yourself Regularly

Getting on a scale is something that many people avoid as it can be painful and disappointing if you are overweight. However, weighing yourself on a regular basis is an important tool to maintain a healthy lifestyle and can be a powerful motivator for healthy living. To better explain this, I like to share my possum analogy with my patients.

We used to have a possum that patrolled our backyard each night. It seemed harmless enough, but the kids weren't really excited about having an animal that resembled a rat in our backyard. I did some research and learned that light was one of the best ways to keep the possum off our property. Well, weight is sort of like a possum. Shining the light of your eyes on the scale and seeing how much you weigh helps to keep the extra pounds away.

Unfortunately, as I learned the hard way many years ago, it's easy to slowly gain weight without realizing it. Checking your weight on a regular basis means you're likely to catch things before you have a big problem. If you find your weight creeping upward, you will be able to make small changes to your diet and exercise routine so that you don't continue to gain weight. Without weighing yourself, you may have no idea that you have a problem until your clothes don't fit. At that point, you may have gained fifteen to twenty pounds, or even more than that.

I recommend that you weigh yourself at the same time of day at least once per week. Most people prefer weigh-ins first thing in the morning because you can incorporate this as a part of your morning routine. Studies have also shown that keeping a record of your weight helps keep you on track. One easy way to do this is to use a digital scale—such as the FitBit Aria or the digital scale from Withings—that records your weight and also provides a reasonably accurate measure of body fat). If you don't already have a scale, it's a worthwhile investment.

Habit 13: Automate Eating

In previous habits, I've alluded to the idea of automating your healthy eating program. Habit 13 provides strategies to help automate your food choices to make it as easy as possible to eat and drink foods rich in nutrients and in line with your calorie goals. This frees you up to think about other important parts of your life.

Think about where and when you eat most of your meals and create a plan to ensure you have convenient, healthy choices for each meal. If you decide that oatmeal and fruit would be a good healthy breakfast, make that an automatic part of your morning by ensuring that oatmeal and fruit are readily available. Similarly, avoid having to figure out what to eat for dinner when you get home. Your best bet is to have healthy options ready to go so it's easier to make good choices. Automation means that your home (and other places where you spend significant time) is stocked with the foods that you have chosen to be a part of your healthy eating plan. If you travel or frequently enjoy restaurants, spend time reviewing on-line menus so you have good choices for eating healthy wherever you are. Keep in mind that automation can lead to unhealthy eating if you make the wrong foods readily available. The key is to make eating healthy foods convenient and easy.

Some say that eating in this way is boring and lacks spontaneity. My response is that it works. If healthy foods are convenient, then you will eat them more consistently. Planning your food choices ensures that you avoid situations where you are famished and likely to make poor food choices. Automation is very important to successfully reach and maintain an optimal weight and optimal wellness. Planning meals in advance is a helpful tool to optimize your chances for nutritional success.

◈ ◈ ◈

Angelina is a 57 year old dental hygienist whose 30 pound weight gain resulted in a variety of different medical problems. Angelina never stepped on a scale except at the doctor's office and hadn't noticed her gradual weight gain.

Angelina told me her busy schedule didn't allow time for lunch. As a result, she snacked on about four candy bars per day to get through each work day. She was shocked to realize that she was getting about 800-1000 calories each day from candy bars, which was half of her recommended daily calorie goal.

Angelina was receptive to the idea of automating her lunch and snacks to ensure that she satiates her hunger while meeting her nutritional goals. Angelina settled on a pre-packaged healthy salad as her standard lunch and apples as her main snack food. Quick calculations confirmed that these foods were in line with her daily calorie goal, as well as her other nutritional goals. Angelina arranged to purchase a week's worth of these foods every Sunday and agreed to stock her office refrigerator so she would be able to automate her daytime eating without having to resort to a candy bar.

Angelina was happy as this simple step made her life less stressful and provided a clear roadmap to lose the excess weight she had been carrying for years. Six months later, Angelina called to tell me that automating her meals was working. Angelina had more energy and had lost fifteen pounds. As she had found other healthy lunch and snack options to add more variety to her meals, she was optimistic that this would work for the long-term.

❖ ❖ ❖

Habit 14: Slow Down

Slowing down is a simple but profound tactic to avoid overeating and overconsuming calories. It turns out that the faster you eat, the more you eat. In one study, researchers found that people ate more calories when they had ten minutes to eat as compared to having thirty minutes to eat. When you eat quickly, you don't have time to think about hunger or whether you are already full. When you slow down the eating process, you actually tend to eat less.

It takes about twenty minutes after you start to eat for your brain to sense that you're getting full. If you eat an entire meal in ten minutes (the duration of the average American meal), your brain won't have time to sense that you're full and send signals to stop eating. By eating so quickly, you're responding to the taste of the food or just to the fact that there is still food left on your plate rather than what your body truly needs. On the other hand, if you slow down, you begin to gain a better awareness of your internal cues indicating you've eaten enough and it's time to stop.

There are a number of simple ways to slow down the eating process. Focus your attention on thoroughly chewing your food, cutting food into small pieces, and eating one piece at a time. One study found that participants ate 30% fewer calories when using chopsticks because chopsticks tend to slow down the eating process. If you slow down and take at least twenty minutes to eat each meal, it's easier to control your portions and keep your daily calorie intake in line. I call this the "twenty minute rule."

―――――――――◈ ◈ ◈―――――――――

Maria is a 44 years old store manager who lost twenty pounds over the past year by making better food choices and becoming more active. However, Maria is frustrated that she cannot drop the stubborn last fifteen pounds to get to her goal weight. Despite eating healthy food, Maria eats quickly. Typically, Maria plows through her lunch of a large turkey sandwich, a plate of melon, and also a cup of almonds in about three minutes. Similarly, Maria usually eats dinner in about five minutes in between helping her kids with their schoolwork.

Maria and I reviewed her food choices and found that her large portion sizes meant her calorie counts were significantly higher than they should be. She was really frustrated because she had been trying her best to make good food choices. However, her habit of eating an entire meal so quickly meant that she wasn't focusing on how much food her body needs. In fact, her body never had time to determine if her hunger had been satisfied because she finished eating before her body could signal to her that she was full.

Maria agreed to use a timer to ensure that she spent at least twenty minutes on each meal. She also agreed to eat without the distraction of watching TV or using her tablet or smartphone. Maria called me a month later and shared that taking extra time to eat helped her stop eating when her hunger had been satisfied—and she was eating a lot less food this way. She had lost five pounds so far and was gaining confidence that she could reach her goal weight.

❖ ❖ ❖

Habit 15: Avoid Excessive Alcohol

You may have read in other books that drinking a moderate amount of alcohol each day, especially red wine, is a healthy practice. Unfortunately, I have to tell you that there are numerous reasons why consuming more than occasional alcohol does not promote wellness.

In September of 2015, a study about the health effects of alcohol was published in the highly respected medical journal *The Lancet*. This study involved 115,000 patients in 12 different countries and found that heavy alcohol use was associated with a 31-54% increased risk of death, mostly due to increased cancer risk. Interestingly, researchers found a direct correlation between the risk of cancer and the amount of alcohol consumption. The greater the alcohol use, the greater the likelihood of cancer. The researchers did note a reduction in heart attack risk associated with drinking wine, but found that this benefit was greatly offset by the increased cancer risk. In particular, alcohol was found to increase the risk of cancers of the mouth, esophagus, stomach, colon, liver, breast, ovaries, head, and neck.

Alcohol has other negative effects on the body. Alcohol significantly reduces both the quantity and quality of sleep. Anything that detrimentally affects sleep should be minimized or avoided as sufficient sleep is critical to good health. Second, alcohol is a source of empty calories. In a nation where two-thirds of people are overweight or obese, keeping a close watch on calorie consumption is extremely important. Reducing calories by 100 calories per day (about the amount in one small glass of wine or one light beer) will result in about ten pounds of weight loss over the course of a year. Finally, in addition to increasing the risk of many cancers, alcohol also increases the risk of other health problems including acid reflux, ulcers, liver failure, and high blood pressure.

Because of all these reasons, I recommend avoiding excessive alcohol. You may want to have an occasional glass of wine, but regular consumption of alcohol isn't something that I recommend. When my patients reduce their consumption of alcohol, they often note how much better they sleep and how much more energetic they feel. They also find it's much easier to reach and maintain their ideal weight.

Think about the role that alcohol plays in your life. Read some of the articles and studies about alcohol listed in the reference section of this book. Take an honest look at the role that alcohol plays in your life and decide whether this is a habit that you want to address during one of your monthly four-column exercises.

Habit 16: Practice Regular Physical Activity

I don't think it comes as much of a surprise that one of main habits of *The Wellness Code* is to get more physical activity. Study after study has shown that a sedentary, inactive lifestyle is a major risk factor for a variety of medical problems such as heart disease, osteoporosis, high blood pressure, sleep issues, and various types of cancer.

Being active is crucial to your health. In addition to the physical payoffs of exercise, there are also many mental and emotional benefits. Exercise boosts memory, concentration, happiness, and discipline and reduces anxiety levels and other forms of stress. Of course, before starting or changing any exercise program, please review the specifics of any activity plan with your personal physician or healthcare provider to see what's safe and optimal for you.

Sadly, over the last twenty-five years, the average person has become less active. In general, we tend to drive rather than walk, take the elevator instead of the stairs, and send an email or text instead of walk down the hall to talk with a coworker or family member.

The average American gets about 4,000-5,000 steps per day while the generally accepted goal for a healthy person is get at least 10,000 steps per day. To put this in perspective, 2,000 steps is roughly equivalent to about one mile and burns about 100 calories. When I tell folks to take 10,000 steps per day, the response is typically a facial grimace that lets me know that this is not likely to happen. However, it's not nearly as tough as it seems.

The first step (no pun intended) in becoming more active is to determine if you're getting a sufficient number of steps each day. For most people, the best way to monitor steps is a fitness tracker. Keeping track of your steps can provide an indicator to see if you are getting enough activity.

A Stanford University study found that those who used a fitness tracker had better blood pressure readings and were more successful at losing weight. The researchers reviewed 26 studies involving over 2,700 patients and found that those who used a fitness tracker were 27% more active. This translated to walking about an extra mile each day. The study also found that setting a goal of about 10,000 steps per day was a strong predictor of increased physical activity.

There are many options available for fitness tracking, so you can easily find something that fits your budget and your lifestyle. Options now range from classic clip-on devices to fitness trackers that are worn on the wrist. For those who don't like to wear a device, there are apps for the iPhone and Android to track your steps. Some of these apps also estimate how many calories you burn. Another benefit of this technology is that you see your results in real-time, which can provide motivation to become more active. For example, if it's 6 p.m. and you see that you've only taken about 5,000 steps so far that day, you might be motivated to go for a walk instead of sitting on the couch to watch your favorite television show.

When you start monitoring your steps, spend the first few days measuring how many steps you average per day. Once you have an idea of your typical steps per day, speak with your physician to create a safe, realistic plan for increasing your activity. In general, I recommend taking 10,000 total steps per day, but it's not always realistic to immediately transition from your current activity level to 10,000 steps a day. It often works better to gradually increase your daily steps in increments of 1,000. If you are currently walking 5,000 steps per day, then your new goal would be to take 6,000 steps per day. Once you're comfortable getting 6,000 steps per day, then the next goal would be 7,000 steps per day, and so on.

Make this process fun and you will be more likely to reach your activity goal. Remember linkage? Consider ways to link activities that you enjoy with walking. Schedule walks with a friend or colleague if possible.

However you measure your daily steps, be sure to find a way to track your activity over time. This allows you to take a look back and see your progress. Many fitness apps and trackers will store historical information to make this easy. It turns out that documenting and reviewing the number of steps that you get per day significantly increases the chances that you'll succeed with your activity plan.

$$\diamond \diamond \diamond$$

Patricia is a 36 year old nurse who was frustrated with her struggles to lose weight. When she was younger, she simply ate less if she noticed that she'd put on a couple of pounds and the weight came right off. However, this no longer worked. Over the past several years, her weight had drifted up to 150 pounds. Patricia realized that she needed to become more active to boost her metabolism. Unfortunately, Patricia's job was largely sedentary—mostly involving sitting at a desk—and she didn't enjoy exercise. With good intentions, Patricia had purchased a fancy elliptical trainer over a year ago, but had used it only a few times. I suggested to Patricia that linkage might help her find a way to enjoy exercising and asked her to brainstorm to find an activity she could link to exercise. When Patricia mentioned how much she enjoys watching the TV show *Modern Family*, I suggested that she make it a rule that she could only watch *Modern Family* while she exercised on her elliptical trainer. Patricia agreed to give this a try.

A month later, Patricia came back to see me and she looked like a different person. She had lost seven pounds and had a vibrant look in her eyes. She told me she was exercising daily and had already gone back and watched just about every episode of *Modern Family*. Patricia was now moving on to watch her other favorite sitcoms, and was excited to get up each morning looking forward to exercising for the first time in her life. Because she linked exercise to watching her favorite TV show, what had been a chore had become something she looked forward to doing.

◈ ◈ ◈

If possible, try using a fitness tracker—either the clip-on variety or one worn on the wrist. Another option is to use a fitness tracking app. Measure how many steps you take each day and then meet with your doctor to set your activity goals.

Habit 17: The Importance of Aerobic Exercise

Habit 16 of *The Wellness Code* emphasized the importance of being active and keeping track of how many steps you take each day. After making sure that you're getting the correct number of steps each day, the second step in any activity plan is to get the optimal amount of aerobic exercise each week.

Examples of aerobic exercise include power walking, using an elliptical trainer, biking, or swimming. Please discuss the specifics of your exercise program with your personal physician to see what would be safe and effective for you. For most patients, I recommend twenty to thirty minutes of aerobic exercise five days a week. Using a fitness tracker increases the likelihood that you will be consistent with your exercise program. Many fitness trackers can monitor aerobic exercise, in addition to total steps. There are also apps that use GPS to monitor your walks, runs, hikes, or bike rides.

The first step is to pick an exercise program that is the right fit for you. After getting a list of your doctor's approved activities for exercise, think through which ones you are most likely to stick with in the long term. The activity you choose should be fun and fit into your current lifestyle. For me, it is an elliptical trainer. I love my elliptical trainer as I can watch TV shows, movies, or music concerts on my tablet or smartphone while I exercise. What works best for you? What are you most likely to enjoy and stick with for the long-term?

Once you decide, make a plan to put exercise on your schedule. Schedule exercise just like you would a meeting or a dinner or anything else that's a priority for you. Make exercise a planned part of your day and your week. For most, the best time to exercise is first thing in the morning so you don't get sidetracked and not exercise at all. However, the best time for others may be midday or in the evening. Figure out the best time of day for you and your schedule. Then block off your calendar for your exercise appointment. Telling someone else about your new exercise plan significantly increases the likelihood that you will stick with your plan. A public statement of your plans can support your motivation and commitment to exercise.

I'm often asked how many calories are burned during each type of exercise or activity. This chart provides a list of estimated calories burned for one hour of various activities.

Calories Burned for Various Activities

Activity	Weight of Person and Calories Burned		
(1 hour duration)	160 lbs.	200 lbs.	240 lbs.
Aerobics, low impact	365	455	545
Aerobics, water	402	501	600
Basketball game	584	728	872
Bicycling, < 10 mph, leisure	292	364	436
Bowling	219	273	327
Canoeing	256	319	382
Dancing, ballroom	219	273	327
Elliptical trainer, moderate effort	365	455	545
Football, touch or flag	584	728	872
Golfing, carrying clubs	314	391	469
Hiking	438	546	654
Ice skating	511	637	763
Racquetball	511	637	763
Resistance (weight) training	365	455	545
Rollerblading	548	683	818
Rowing, stationary	438	546	654
Running, 5 mph	606	755	905
Skiing, cross-country	496	619	741
Skiing, downhill	314	391	469
Softball or baseball	365	455	545
Stair treadmill	657	819	981
Swimming laps, light or moderate	423	528	632
Tennis, singles	584	728	872
Volleyball	292	364	436
Walking, 3.5 mph	314	391	469
Yoga, hatha	183	228	273

Adapted from: Ainsworth BE, et al. 2011 compendium of physical activities: A second update of codes and MET values. Medicine & Science in Sports & Exercise. 2011;43:1575.

As you can see, it is difficult to burn a significant number of calories which is why keeping calorie intake in line is so important. In addition, many websites, such as MyFitnessPal.com, have calculators where you can enter in basic information to calculate calories burned.

———◈ ◈ ◈———

Sandra is a 45 year old stay-at-home mom who told me she was having trouble exercising on a regular basis. Despite being diagnosed with breast cancer and her oncologist emphasizing to her how important regular exercise is for her recovery, Sandra had difficulty "finding time" to exercise, despite the fact that she owned a treadmill. Sandra and I discussed the importance of scheduling time to exercise, telling others about her plan to exercise, and linking pleasurable activities to exercise such as reading her favorite magazine and going on Facebook. Sandra agreed to exercise daily and tell her husband that she planned to get on the treadmill for a minimum of twenty minutes each day. To ensure this happened, she planned to exercise first thing in the morning before her kids woke up. A few months later, Sandra called me and let me know she was exercising on her treadmill five times per week. Practicing this important habit was a huge step in the right direction for Sandra.

———◈ ◈ ◈———

Habit 18: Weight Training

In habit 16 and habit 17, I reviewed the importance of being active and practicing consistent aerobic exercise. However, one commonly overlooked aspect of exercise is weight training. Weight training adds tremendous value above and beyond running on a treadmill, using an elliptical trainer, or swimming.

Weight training is an important habit because it helps build muscle, which is the prime driver of metabolism. In general, the more muscle mass you have, the more calories you burn, which helps control weight. In addition to building muscle and helping maintain your weight, weight training also helps maintain the strength of your bones. This is a particular concern for women, who are at greater risk for osteoporosis. However, osteoporosis can also be an issue for men. In addition, certain medications, such as proton pump inhibitors used for acid reflux, increase the risk of bone loss and osteoporosis.

When I say weight training, you may envision bench pressing large amounts of weights in a sweaty gym, but there are many ways to add resistance training to your routine. Sometimes simple weight resistance tools are already present on elliptical machines, treadmills or stationary bikes.

When you begin a weight training program, be sure to do so safely in consultation with your healthcare provider and possibly a personal trainer. A personal trainer can help ensure that your technique is correct. Incorrectly lifting weights can actually do more harm than good as a strained muscle can derail your exercise program for significant periods of time. If necessary, use a spotter. Weight training two to three times per week can be a pivotal part of a healthy exercise program

Kathleen is a 54 year old patient who came to see me as a new patient. She takes a "statin" medication for high cholesterol and an 81 mg aspirin each day. She exercises at a gym five times per week and eats mostly vegetables and lean protein. She also attends a yoga class twice weekly and recently started meditating ten minutes a day.

I reviewed her old medical records and noticed a bone density scan from six months ago showed osteopenia or bones that are thinner than normal. Kathleen said that her previous doctor recommended rechecking the scan in two years. I ordered some blood tests and found that Kathleen's vitamin D level was significantly below the normal range. I recommended that Kathleen take a vitamin D supplement to get her level into the optimal range.

I pointed out that Kathleen's exercise routine focused mostly on aerobic exercise and stretching, but was deficient in terms of weight lifting. Kathleen laughed and said that she hadn't thought of lifting weights. We discussed that a weight training routine is one of the most important things she could do to improve the strength of her bones.

After our appointment, Kathleen spoke with a trainer at her gym and they designed a weekly weight training regimen for her. They also found ways to add low-level resistance training to her aerobic exercise program and her yoga program. I was extremely impressed with how motivated Kathleen was to change her routine. Two years later, we rechecked another bone density scan and, fortunately, her bone strength had improved.

◆ ◆ ◆

Habit 19: Stretch

Another often neglected aspect of an optimal activity program is stretching. For many people, stretching is not a priority as it isn't as exciting as aerobic exercise and doesn't provide the visible results of weight lifting. With busy schedules, stretching often doesn't even make it onto weekly to-do lists. However, I would argue that stretching is just as important to an optimal exercise regimen as the other forms of exercise.

Stretching has some key features that make it distinctly beneficial. First, stretching helps prevent injuries. You cannot be consistent with aerobic exercise or weight training if you have muscle pulls and other injuries. If you talk to any personal trainer, you will learn how important stretching is to prevent injuries, especially as you get older and your muscles and tendons don't respond quite as well as in younger days.

In addition, stretching adds a different form of exercise to your regimen. This is because stretching is actually a form of meditation. Meditation is simply where you focus on a word, phrase, or movement for an extended period of time and release your conscious thoughts to stay focused on the word, phrase, or movement. We will explore meditation is more detail in habit 20 of *The Wellness Code*, but stretching can be a powerful meditative tool. For example, let's say that you're stretching your lower leg muscles with each stretch lasting for twenty seconds. As you perform that gentle stretch, place your focus and attention on the stretch and then release your conscious thoughts as they arise in your mind. Passively release each thought as it enters your mind and return your focus to the stretch. This allows stretching to improve your flexibility while also providing the benefits of meditation that I will discuss in habit 20.

Think of ways to make stretching a part of your regular routine. Ideally, stretch before you begin your exercise routine. However, it can also be done at any time of day. It's great to stretch when you first wake in the morning to get your muscle loosened up for the day. It can also be done before sleep to get your body relaxed. A good starting point is to simply add five minutes of stretching to your day.

◆ ◆ ◆

Alex is a 45 year old patient of mine who is an orthopedic surgeon at a local hospital. Alex is married and has two young children. He takes extremely good care of himself by running for thirty minutes five days a week and also lifts weights twice per week. Alex tells me that exercise has always helped him relax and control his stress. However, he came to see me because he's finding it more and more difficult to handle all of his responsibilities and he has started to suffer from insomnia because of the stress. Alex didn't want to consider a medication at this time and said that he's looking for a lifestyle change that might help. I brought up several tools to help with stress management. Alex was open to the idea of meditation. However, he said he's never been able to sit still long enough to meditate.

I suggested that Alex add a daily stretching routine and use that as a portal to practice meditation. As soon as I mentioned this, I could see a light bulb go off in his head. He told me years ago he attended a yoga class to help control his stress when his father was undergoing some serious medical problems. Alex said that he remembers feeling much better after each yoga class so he agreed to begin a daily stretching routine. A few weeks later, Alex reported to me that this new program was helping a great deal and that he was finding it easier to handle the stresses of daily living. He said that the daily stretching was helping him feel more centered and content with his life.

◆ ◆ ◆

Habit 20: Meditate

If I told you that a recent study showed that performing one specific activity each day would reduce your risk of dying by 48%, would you give it a try? I'm guessing your answer is probably "yes."

Well, that's what I'll be discussing in this habit of *The Wellness Code*. It's something that is so simple and yet is vitally important to your health. In previous habits, I discussed the importance of physical activity, aerobic exercise, weight training, and stretching. In this habit, I'll be explaining the importance of moving less. Yes, less. Human bodies are peculiar things in that it's beneficial to both to move more and to move less. Getting sufficient physical activity helps to keep your body "in shape." However, you also need short periods of time each day for your mind to take a break. This is time for you to turn off your brain and allow it to recharge.

The brain is a powerful organ that can process loads of information and formulate spectacular ideas. However, for the mind to work optimally, it needs short breaks; periods of time where it can reboot and restore itself to optimal functioning. If you don't give your mind these short breaks, stress will build up within you and eventually result in significant health problems. Stress weakens your immune system and increases the likelihood that illness will develop in the areas of your body where you already have a health vulnerability. Thus, this can affect your intestinal system, cardiovascular system, musculoskeletal system, or other parts of your body. It is critically important to take care of your mind and ensure that you're able to effectively handle stress before it handles you.

Each night, I charge my smartphone so that it has a full battery when I wake up in the morning. Well, one day I fell asleep and forgot to charge my phone and I woke in the morning to find that I was starting my day with a phone with a dead battery.

I realized this is a good analogy for life. You need to use your mind and body throughout the day. However, if you don't recharge your "batteries," eventually you'll wake up one morning with a "dead battery." This can be experienced as just a lack of energy or as a potentially serious health problem.

One of the best ways to recharge your batteries is meditation. Meditation is a period of time each day when you turn off your conscious thoughts and allow your mind to take a short break and recharge. It's difficult to not have a conscious thought, so one of the most effective ways to meditate is to focus on something. It can be your breath, a body movement, or a mantra (a word or phrase on which you focus).

Dr. Herbert Benson of Harvard Medical School has published studies where he showed that one of the most effective meditative practices is to find a word or phrase that holds deep meaning to the meditator. It could be the name of someone special, a religious passage, or anything that holds special meaning for you. Dr. Benson found that people get better results from meditation by focusing on a word or phrase that holds personal meaning rather than focusing on a generic word such as peace or love.

The next step is to find a quiet place to sit down where you'll be free of distractions and noise. With eyes either open or closed, repeat your focus word or phrase either out loud or to yourself. You will probably find that after about twenty seconds, thoughts will enter your mind (such as, "Why am I doing nothing right now?"). When this happens, let those thoughts go and gently return to your focus word or phrase.

Meditating is sort of like driving a car. As you're driving, the car might shift a bit to the right or left in your lane. When this happens, you gently turn the steering wheel to keep the car going straight. Likewise, your goal is to keep your mind on your focus word or phrase. When your mind starts to wander and think about other things, passively let the thought go and return to your focus word or phrase. This is a process of training your mind to stay focused without conscious thought. Meditation is a true vacation for the mind.

Turning off your conscious mind allows for the healing of your mind and body. Some call this meditation. Some calls this simple relaxation. Dr. Benson calls it The Relaxation Response. No matter what it is called, it is a rewarding process that makes every other minute of the day that much better.

For new meditators, I usually recommend starting with two minutes a day. Once you have been able to consistently meditate for two minutes a day, try to increase the sessions to a five minute session each day. Once you get more comfortable with meditation, you can gradually increase the duration of your sessions with an ultimate goal of twenty minutes per day. Don't worry if this is difficult for you as meditation is one of the most challenging habits in *The Wellness Code*. Be patient with yourself and stick with it even if your meditation sessions are brief.

A recent study detailed the health benefits of meditation and those benefits were impressive. In this study, patients were randomized to either meditation on a consistent basis or attending a health education course. The researchers found that after five years, the patients who meditated had a 48% lower risk of death, heart attack, and stroke when compared to those who attended the health education classes. That's a staggering number. If a medication could give people that much benefit, it would likely become one of the biggest selling pharmaceutical products of all-time. Happily, you can achieve this benefit from a basic habit that can be practiced every day without the need for a prescription or expensive equipment.

What about other relaxation techniques such as yoga, Pilates, biofeedback, or other techniques? Each of these can be helpful as well. The key is to find a relaxation technique where you practice focusing your attention on a word, phrase, or movement for a period of time and then passively let your thoughts go when thoughts arise in your mind. Many people are amazed by how much better they feel when they start practicing the discipline of meditation.

Joanne is a 33 year old financial executive with a history of elevated triglyceride levels and asthma. She had her first child two years ago, which motivated her to take better care of herself. Before becoming a parent, she ate a lot of fast food and didn't exercise often. However, having a child made her think more seriously about her health. She started to exercise at the gym six days a week, carefully watch her diet, and get sufficient restorative sleep each night. Joanne saw me for a physical and all of her screening tests, including her blood tests, were perfect. Her vital signs were also excellent and no problems were found on her evaluation.

Whenever I see a patient for a checkup, we try to find at least one new healthy habit to work on and Joanne asked me which habit she should address this year. Based on her patient history, I noted that she reported being under a lot of stress at home and at work so I asked her to try adding a meditation practice to her daily regimen. As Joanne didn't have time to join a meditation group, I suggested she download a meditation app and give that a try. Joanne tried a meditation app called *Calm* and she called me a few weeks later to let me know two things. First, she said that meditation was incredibly difficult for her. She said that her active mind was tough to tame and that sitting still for a few minutes was a challenge for her, but she was still trying her best to practice this every day. She also noted that she was sleeping a lot better and that she felt a lot calmer at work which she attributed to the mediation practice. Joanne said she was excited to see such impressive results so quickly and that she planned to continue this practice into the future.

————————————— ◈ ◈ ◈ —————————————

If you've never meditated before, try it for just two minutes a day. The best way to start is to pick a short word or phrase with which you connect on a positive, personal level. Sit in a comfortable chair and slowly repeat the word or phrase to yourself for two minutes. When other thoughts try to intrude into your mind (which usually happens after about twenty seconds), let those thoughts go and then return to the repetition. This simple technique can be extremely healing. If you'd like to try an app to help you, there are many excellent meditation apps including *Calm*, *The Mindfulness App*, and *Headspace*.

Habit 21: Plan Your Calendar Weekly

Planning your schedule is important to make sure that the activities that fill up your days reflect your priorities and values. Thus, you should spend time on activities that strengthen the important relationships in your life and bring joy to your life. If you don't prioritize these activities, you may find that your schedule fills up with less meaningful things.

Many people focus on the urgent demands of daily life at the expense of truly important activities and relationships. These priorities include close ties to friends and family, a good healthy relationship with your spouse or partner, exercise, proper nutrition, and a consistent stress reduction practice. These are essential to your health, but they only happen when you prioritize them and plan your schedule to include them. Good intentions tend to fall by the wayside when you get busy.

When life gets busy, you may skip some of these important activities for a few days. This can easily become a couple of weeks, which can turn into a month or two. Before you realize it, a year has passed and you've forgotten all about your good intentions. This is why a schedule is so important to your health.

Each week, plan your schedule. By that, I mean schedule your entire week down to when you'll exercise, when you'll see your friends and family and when you'll practice your favorite hobby.

Daily planning is important for listing things that need to be taken care of each day. Monthly, quarterly, and annual reviews of your schedule also have a role in long-term goal setting. However, a week is the ideal mid-level time period that allows for both short term and long term views of your life.

Maintain your schedule in a way that is convenient and portable. For most, a digital scheduler is best, but an old-fashioned paper schedule works as well. Review your schedule at least once each week. Plan out everything that you want to accomplish that week and make sure that you are available for each appointment that you schedule.

Be sure to schedule activities such as exercise, time with your children, time with friends, time to practice your hobbies, time to watch your favorite TV show, and time to have dinner with your spouse or partner. Emergencies happen and your schedule may need to be adjusted as you proceed through the week, but the goal here is to at least have everything "booked" before the week starts to maximize your chances of accomplishing what you hope to get done.

If your schedule impacts others in your family, it's also important to keep a central schedule so that everyone can stay informed about upcoming events. We have a huge paper calendar hanging on the wall in our kitchen. The calendar is color-coded so each family member can quickly tell which activity applies to which person. Doctor's appointments, sports practices, upcoming tests and work events all get recorded on this wall calendar. The family calendar is another way to ensure everyone stays connected to one another.

◈ ◈ ◈

Tom is a 45 year old chiropractor who came to see me because his nurse recently checked his blood pressure and found it was elevated. He's never had any significant health issues, so this was a surprise for him and got his attention. Tom was extremely well versed in the principles of a healthy lifestyle. In fact, he lectured on nutrition, stress management, and how exercise can help common musculoskeletal problems like arthritis, fibromyalgia, and minor sports injuries. As we discussed all of this, it became clear to me that Tom certainly didn't have an issue in terms of knowledge.

However, he also told me that he didn't always practice what he preaches. He said that his office practice was extremely busy and his family life was also hectic, so he didn't have the time to take good care of himself. He said that over the past year, he has rarely exercised and frequently eats takeout restaurant food. He also said that his sleep habits have become poor as he finds himself doing office-related paperwork late at night, and then getting up early in the morning to start seeing patients.

Because of all this, he has gained twenty-five pounds in the last couple of years. I checked his blood pressure and confirmed that it was elevated. In fact, it was so elevated that I prescribed a blood pressure lowering medication that day. I also mentioned that his lifestyle and his weight gain may be contributing to his high blood pressure. Tom said that he'd love to take better care of himself, but he simply doesn't have the time to make it happen.

Tom and I then spent an hour reviewing his weekly schedule. We literally went through his calendar hour by hour and found that he was spending a lot of time doing things that should be delegated to his office staff. I also found that he spends ninety minutes a day going out to lunch rather than bringing in something healthy that he can eat at the office.

By reviewing his calendar, we found about 2-3 hours each day that could be used for better lifestyle practices. We again reviewed his calendar and added in these lifestyle practices, including exercise and meditation. We literally scheduled these activities as appointments on Tom's calendar. We also took the step to schedule his bedtime to ensure that he would get 7-8 hours of continuous sleep each night. We spoke about the fact that urgent issues will come up and he should strive to be flexible with his schedule.

Tom left the office that day with a clearly planned weekly calendar that made it realistic for him to take good care of himself. He returned to see me a month later with a big smile on his face as he was proud that he had generally stuck with the schedule for the entire month. His schedule required a bit of tweaking, but it was working to help him stay on target. In addition, his blood pressure was under much better control.

◈ ◈ ◈

Be sure to plan your calendar each week. Most people do their calendar planning on Sunday, but pick a day of the week that works to plan your weekly calendar. Make this a regular practice. You may also want to review your plans with your closest family members and friends to make sure everything is coordinated. Have fun with this. The rewards will be tremendous.

Habit 22: Practice Good Dental Hygiene

I am including dental care as a habit because dental health does relate to overall health and longevity. Disorders of the teeth lead to inflammation and this inflammation can be damaging to the rest of the body. In fact, inflammation is believed to be a contributing factor to many diseases including autoimmune disorders, coronary heart disease, and some cancers.

There are three essential steps to maintaining healthy teeth:

Step 1: Floss every day. Ideally you should floss after each meal, but be sure to floss at least once per day. Flossing is a great way to remove food particles that get lodged between the teeth and prevent tooth decay.

Step 2: Use a toothpaste with fluoride. We know that fluoride reduces the risk of cavities and thus reduces inflammation. If you're someone who suffers from occasional canker sores (those annoying sores that some people get inside the mouth), please look for toothpaste that does not contain the foaming agent called sodium laurel sulfate (SLS). SLS appears to be one of the most common causes of canker sores. If this is an issue for you, try toothpaste without SLS for a couple of months and see this helps. Fortunately, there are many brands of toothpaste made without SLS including some of the products from Biotene, Sensodyne, and Squigle. If you suffer from canker sores, be sure to check the ingredient label to make sure your toothpaste is free of SLS.

Step 3: Chew a piece of sugarless gum after meals. Chewing gum increases saliva production and this helps to naturally cleanse and protect the teeth from inflammation. In addition, Xylitol (which is contained in some brands of chewing gum and toothpaste) is a natural product that appears to prevent cavities by interfering with bacteria's ability to attach to the teeth and cause cavities. In some studies, Xylitol has proven to be equal to, or even better than, fluoride in preventing cavities. The one downside I should mention is that too much Xylitol can lead to bowel irregularities such as diarrhea. If this is an issue, your consumption of Xylitol may need to be reduced or eliminated. Most people should limit their daily consumption of Xylitol to no more than six to ten grams.

Make flossing, brushing with a fluoride toothpaste (without sodium laurel sulfate), and chewing a piece of sugarless Xylitol gum part of your daily routine.

◈ ◈ ◈

Craig is a 52 year old contractor who came to see me (accompanied by his wife) because his frequent nighttime awakenings had become a big problem in recent years. Craig was exhausted and said he felt he never got a good night's sleep.

Craig's wife said he's not snoring, so that eliminated a number of potential causes for Craig's sleep issues. I asked Craig to describe his nightly routine and what he remembers about his nighttime awakenings. Craig mentioned that he frequently wakes up during the night because of his dry mouth and he can't get back to sleep. He also told me he drinks water when he wakes up in the middle of the night with a dry mouth. Craig gets up about every two hours each night, drinks water, and goes to the bathroom. When people get up this often during the night, they aren't able to achieve sufficient deep, restorative sleep which is needed to feel refreshed. I suggested to Craig that his dry mouth problem seemed to be contributing to his sleep issues.

I told Craig to try using a dry mouth toothpaste and mouthwash each night. My hope was that improving his dry mouth would improve his sleep patterns. I also asked Craig to avoid food and beverages two hours before bedtime. A few weeks later, Craig reported that he felt much better during the day, In particular, his fatigue had lifted and his energy level had returned to normal. Craig told me that using the new toothpaste and mouthwash enabled him to stop drinking water at night and he no longer had to get up at night to urinate. Thus, his sleep quality was much improved. Craig said that these small changes had a very large impact in the quality and quantity of his sleep.

◈ ◈ ◈

Habit 23: Practice Safe Driving Habits

When I talk to patients about their driving habits, I usually see one of those knowing head nods. We all know that safe driving habits are crucial in this day and age. We also know that the quality of driving has been declining for years and there are many reasons for this.

The 24-hour news and life cycle has taken multitasking to a whole new level. Some choose to text during many different activities: while having dinner, crossing the street, and even when driving. Some individuals have forgotten that texting requires a proper place and time to stay safe.

It used to be that the music on the radio and a conversation with a passenger were the main distractions in a car. However, with the advent of smartphones, tablets, GPS gadgets and a host of other items, the list of distractions has grown exponentially.

I remember as a child watching my father try to control my brother and me while he drove down the highway and marveling at how much he was able to do while he drove. However, that was nothing compared to today. Today I see people drinking coffee, applying makeup, texting their friends, listening to the radio, getting directions on the GPS, and checking Facebook all while trying to calm down their children in the back seat.

A recent study by the Governors Highway Safety Association looked at 350 scientific papers and found that about 20% of all car accidents are linked to smartphone usage. That is close to one in five accidents! That statistic is staggering but true.

Here are some other statistics to think about:

- Texting while driving makes a driver 23 times more likely to crash.
- 1 out of every 4 car accidents in the United States is caused by texting and driving.
- Texting while driving is 6 times more likely to cause an accident than drunk driving.
- Drivers talking on a cell phone are 4 times more likely to have a car accident.
- Texting while driving causes a 400% increase in time spent with eyes off the road.

Here are some statistics about teen drivers:

- 15 to 19 year-olds make up the largest proportion of distracted drivers.
- 11 teens die each day due to texting while driving.
- 21% of teen drivers involved in fatal accidents were distracted by their cell phones.

Many of these accidents cause serious injuries and sometimes even deaths. It is vitally important that people get back to simply focusing on driving. I see some experts recommending hands-free devices, but the truth is that studies have generally shown that hands-free devices still pose some risks. It appears that the primary hazard of using a phone while driving is the loss of focus and attention that speaking on the phone creates. This risk isn't completely eliminated even when using a hands-free device.

My proposal is that you get a bit old-fashioned when it comes to driving. Don't speak on the phone while you drive. Don't use a smartphone or tablet while you drive. If an emergency call comes in or needs to be made, pull over to a safe location. Never text or email while you drive. Don't eat or drink anything while you drive. Focus on keeping your family, your friends, and yourself safe.

You don't need to be connected to electronics all the time. Prior generations somehow survived without all of this technology, so we can go short periods of time without it as well. In fact before around 1990, most people had to use a pay phone to make a call when away from home. Imagine that.

Russell is a 46 year old patient of mine who came to see me for his annual checkup. Russell has been doing well and his medical problems were under good control. His blood pressure was under good control on the medication Losartan (50 mg daily) and his cholesterol was well-controlled on the medication Atorvastatin (40 mg daily). His blood tests looked good, and his physical examination was normal. At the end of his appointment, we discussed healthy habits and he started thinking about picking two habits to practice.

With a smile on his face, Russ quickly picked habit 36 (Love Your Children) as he has three teenagers at home who still need a lot of guidance. He then struggled to select another habit from my list. When he came to the habit of safe driving, he commented that he was worried about his children approaching driving age. I reminded Russell that children learn best through modeling and that one of the most important ways to help his children learn how to drive more safely is for him to model safe, defensive driving habits.

I commented that texting while driving is one of the most dangerous actions a driver can take. I've found that texting while driving is something that few people will admit to doing, but the statistics show that many people engage in this dangerous practice. I told Russell that if texting and driving was an issue for him that he should consider keeping his phone in the back seat or trunk while he drives so he can't access the phone.

Russell's response was, "Well, I think I have a second habit to work on this year." He also said that he planned to discuss safe driving with his children.

———————————◈ ◈ ◈———————————

Make it a priority to not use your smartphone or tablet while you drive. Focus on getting to your destination safe and sound.

Habit 24: Anticipation

It's funny how we learn things from all sorts of interesting places. Sometimes we learn from traditional places like lectures, courses, books, or even online programs. But sometimes we learn important concepts at unexpected times from unexpected sources

If you watched the end of Super Bowl XLIX, you were treated to an incredible ending to an exciting game. In the final minute of the game, the Seattle Seahawks were driving down the field for what looked to be the winning touchdown. They got down to the one-yard line and quarterback Russell Wilson threw a pass into the end zone that was intercepted by Malcolm Butler of the New England Patriots. I watched this game with my children, and we watched the video of the play over and over again. I heard a lot of commentary on why the Seahawks chose to throw the ball rather than run the ball into the end zone. In particular, I heard a lot of folks blaming the coaches for attempting a pass when a running play might have been a safer way to go.

I saw what happened from a different perspective. I saw a defensive football player practicing a habit that I've tried to teach my children for as long as they could listen. This habit is anticipation. If you watch the videotape, you'll see that Malcolm Butler made the interception because he saw the play unfolding and used the information he gathered to anticipate the throw. By anticipating what was happening, he was able to take action, make the interception, and save the game. Though this example was from a football game, anticipation is important in all aspects of life. In particular, it is incredibly important to your health and well-being.

Anticipation is a two-step process: first, pay attention to what's happening and then use your observations to understand what is likely to happen next. Step one happens within yourself—in your mind. Step two is external and involves you taking action based on what you observed in step one. In the case of Super Bowl XLIX, Malcolm Butler observed that Russell Wilson was about to throw the ball into the end zone. Once he made that assessment, he made a break for the ball. He stepped in front of the receiver and intercepted the ball. It was a perfect embodiment of the two step process of anticipation. He displayed observation and action in one perfect play to save the game.

Anticipation is crucial regardless of your profession. The opposite of anticipation is reactivity where you react after things happen to you. Reactivity is a passive process, while anticipation is a proactive process. Anticipation is sensing what is likely to happen and taking necessary action. Anticipation is crucial is all aspects of life, especially healthy living and longevity.

Think about ways that anticipation plays a part in your life and how it can impact your wellness. If your family has a history of certain cancers, do you anticipate that you may be at higher risk to contract cancer and take proactive steps to prevent that from happening? In particular, have you spoken with your health care provider about screening procedures such as a colonoscopy or a mammogram? Do you anticipate activities that could lead to injuries such as skiing or bike riding and find ways to minimize your risks by wearing protective gear? Do you anticipate the dangers of other situations and figure out ways to keep risks in check? On a more practical basis, do you anticipate needing food and household supplies or do you routinely find yourself battling the supermarket lines at 5:30 p.m.?

As you go through your day, think of how you can use anticipation to reduce stress and promote happiness in your life. Use anticipation to your advantage to improve wellness. Observe what's happening around you, and find ways you can take action based on your observations. Take steps to anticipate and avoid health problems by seeing your healthcare provider on a regular basis for check-ups. Anticipation isn't discussed much in books about healthy living, but it's a key concept to grasp and to integrate into your life.

◈ ◈ ◈

Natalie is a 32 year old patient who came to see me because she was experiencing symptoms of diarrhea and nausea. In the past, she rarely had these issues, but lately her symptoms have become more frequent.

She told me that she has a sister with Hashimoto's thyroiditis and a brother with rheumatoid arthritis. I ordered blood and stool tests which were remarkable for a positive titer for anti-endomysial antibodies and tissue transglutaminase antibodies consistent with Celiac disease. Celiac disease is an autoimmune disease where the gluten protein found in wheat, rye, and barley causes an autoimmune reaction in genetically predisposed people. As a result, most breads and pastas are off limits for these patients. In patients with Celiac disease, even a small amount of gluten can trigger a severe autoimmune inflammatory reaction within the intestines. I sent Natalie for further tests with a gastroenterologist including an endoscopy of her upper digestive tract, which confirmed the diagnosis of Celiac disease.

After these tests, Natalie returned to see me to discuss Celiac disease and how to cope with this going forward. Someone with Celiac disease cannot eat any food or product containing gluten. The good news about Celiac disease is that, so long as all gluten is avoided, the illness is generally well-controlled. The bad news is that life with Celiac disease can be challenging. One has to become a gluten detective making sure that gluten isn't present in any food, toothpaste, mouthwash, or supplements. This can be a particular issue at restaurants or at parties or other events.

Anticipation becomes a way of life for people with Celiac disease. I told Natalie that she needs to anticipate meals in a way she never has before. When Natalie goes out to eat, she needs to read the menu carefully and speak with the chef if possible. For example, most soy sauces contain gluten, so all ingredients need to be reviewed as just a tiny bit of gluten can lead to massive inflammation in patients with Celiac disease.

Natalie told me that she's planning to go to her friend's wedding next month and we reviewed how to anticipate and address eating there. She decided to call the caterer in advance to see if gluten-free items would be available. If not, she will plan to bring some options with her. Some beverages, such as beer, have gluten so we also discussed how to anticipate beverage choices as well. Natalie should do well over time and her Celiac disease should be well-controlled so long as she practices active anticipation at home, at work, and during leisure activities.

Anticipation takes some effort, but it is important for everyone as it helps to stay ahead of the game by making sure you take proactive steps to stay healthy in all aspects of your life.

Habit 25: Do Not Smoke

This is a relatively simple habit to discuss, but it's not an easy one to implement. Simply put, smoking is one of the worst things you can do to your body. Smoking increases your risk of heart attack, stroke, and many forms of cancer. It also accelerates the aging process at a staggering rate which is noticeable in the skin of smokers, who often look decades older than they really are. Cigarettes are incredibly addictive, so it can be extremely challenging to quit.

Those who have smoked know that stopping smoking is fraught with challenges and difficulties. Most smokers will say that they know that it's bad for them, but they either feel like they can't stop or they aren't quite ready to stop. I recommend the following four-step process to help you, or someone you know, stop smoking:

1. **Convince the smoker it is crucial to stop smoking**. Smoking increases the risk of many cancers, as well as heart attacks and strokes. It is very important to ensure that the smoker, whether it's you or someone else, understands just how dangerous smoking is the human body.

2. **Help the smoker get ready to stop smoking.** Review the damage that smoking causes and also take into consideration the enjoyment received from smoking. Smokers tend to continue to smoke because they view the short-term pleasure from smoking as outweighing any long-term dangers. Thus, it's important for the smoker to consider the potential pain that may be experienced down the road such as lung disease, hospitalizations, and an early death. When someone truly believes the risks outweigh the benefits, they are ready to begin the process of stopping smoking.

3. **Make a plan to safely and effectively stop smoking.** This should be reviewed with a healthcare provider. The smoker should consider using medication and/or tools, such as hypnosis or meditation, which are now available to help stop smoking. Once the plan is in place, set a quit date.

4. **Develop a long-term plan to not smoke.** Now that the quit date is planned, the smoker should prepare for the quit date to

reduce the chance of a relapse. The average smoker takes seven tries to permanently stop smoking, so it's pivotal that a maintenance plan be in place to ensure the best chance for success. Part of this plan should be for the smoker to know how they will handle stressful life events or even everyday social events. Without a plan, many smokers find themselves reverting back to smoking once they experience the settings or triggers that used to prompt them to smoke. One other factor that improves the success rate of quitting smoking is to have a support system in place. Regardless of whether this support system includes a friend, spouse, co-worker, or a group, having support dramatically increases the odds that the person will be able to successfully break the smoking habit.

The bottom line is that a smoker must find a way to stop smoking—no matter how long it takes. If you're a smoker, make it a goal to stop smoking and persist in that goal until you are successful in quitting. It is worth it for your sake and for the sake of your loved ones. Don't give up! Keep at it. You're worth it! If you know someone who smokes, continue to help this person on their quest to give up smoking. Be patient and understanding and continue to offer help.

Habit 26: Sleep Well

Sleep is something that people sacrifice all too frequently. This is not a good idea as there are significant health benefits to getting enough sleep and significant health problems that stem from insufficient sleep. That's why getting sufficient quality sleep is essential for health and is one of the habits of *The Wellness Code*.

For sleep to be truly restorative, most people need seven to eight continuous hours of sleep per night. Remember that these numbers relate to actual sleep time, not just how long you're in bed. Some people toss and turn or get up and go to the bathroom. Some are woken up frequently throughout the night due to noises, snoring, or body movements such as restless legs. All of these sleep interruptions detract from restorative sleep

In a recent study, men who averaged less than six hours of sleep per night were four times as likely to die over a fourteen year time period. *Yes, they were four times as likely to die.* In another study, people who slept less than six hours per night had a 48% greater risk of developing or dying from heart disease. These are shockingly disturbing numbers.

Insufficient sleep is also related to weight gain. One of the main reasons for this is that people tend to overeat and overindulge in unhealthy foods when sleep deprived.

In some situations, getting insufficient sleep is unavoidable. If a child is ill, a parent may have to stay up much of the night. If a big project is due the next morning, an all-nighter may be in order. However, sleep deprivation should be avoided whenever possible.

Does everyone really need seven to eight hours of sleep each night? With rare exceptions, the answer is yes. There does appear to be a small group of people who only need about five or six hours of sleep per night. However, this is a very small percentage of people so you're probably not one of the lucky few who can get by with very little sleep. If you truly are getting sufficient sleep, you should not need an alarm clock to wake you, you should wake feeling refreshed, and you shouldn't experience daytime sleepiness.

Many of my patients tell me not to worry about their sleep saying, "I already get enough sleep." However, one recent study showed that people tend to overestimate the amount they sleep by 61 minutes each night. This means that people thought they were getting an hour more sleep each night than they really were.

If you suspect you may have a sleep issue, it can be helpful to perform a home sleep evaluation. There are some fairly accurate machines that can be purchased for home use. If you already own a fitness tracker from FitBit, Withings, Basis, Jawbone, Garmin, or Apple, then you already have an easy way to measure your sleep at home. Of course, these home monitoring devices are not nearly as accurate as an evaluation at a sleep lab at a medical facility, but the fitness tracker technology can provide a good general idea of how things are going. One of the biggest benefits that this offers is being able to track your sleep habits over time. The beauty of this is that you can make one change at a time and see how this change impacts your sleep. For example, let's say you're wondering whether your cat is waking you up at night. You can monitor your sleep for a week with the cat in the bedroom and then monitor your sleep for a week with the cat in another room. Having this sort of objective data allows you to carefully assess the impact of each change in lifestyle.

Once you have a good understanding of your current sleep situation, you will know if you are reaching the goal of seven to eight hours of continuous sleep per night. If you're not reaching this goal, these five practical suggestions can often help.

1. Within two hours of going to bed, do not consume any foods or beverages. Most people aren't fully aware of the impact of getting up once or twice each night to go to the bathroom. This is particularly problematic after the age of 50 where an aging bladder can cause such problems. However, even if you don't get out of bed, the feeling of a full bladder can keep you from achieving deep, restorative sleep. Therefore, it's important to follow what I call the "two-hour rule" and set a two hour cut-off time prior to bedtime for eating any foods or drinking any beverages. The key is that your bladder should be empty when you go to bed.

2. Within one hour of bedtime, do not watch TV, use a computer, or use your smartphone. This is what I call the "one-hour rule." That means no email, no internet surfing etc. This may sound difficult but it is achievable. This is important because looking at a TV or computer screen stimulates your brain and body and makes it much more difficult to get quality sleep.

3. Have a regular exercise regimen. Habit 17 explained the importance of regular aerobic exercise. It turns out that regular aerobic exercise is also one of the most important elements of a healthy sleep schedule. It usually works best to exercise in the morning as the stimulation from nighttime exercise can sometimes affect your ability to fall asleep quickly.

4. Have a consistent stress reduction regimen. Isn't it interesting how different habits affect each other? Having a daily stress reduction practice (as discussed in habit 20) can help improve sleep in dramatic ways. Examples include short sessions of yoga, meditation, and Pilates. Unlike aerobic exercise (which should ideally be done in the morning), your relaxation practice can be in the morning or evening (or both).

5. Set a consistent bedtime for yourself. If you don't have a plan of when you need to get to bed each night, it is easy to get caught up in a project or TV show and realize it's late at night and you haven't completed everything you need to do before you go to bed. Do your best to go to bed at the same time each night.

If you're following these five measures and you're still having suboptimal sleep (less than 7-8 hours of continuous sleep), speak with your doctor to see if a referral to a sleep lab might be in order. An overnight sleep evaluation in a sleep lab can be a comprehensive, important way to rule out certain medical problems such as sleep apnea and restless leg syndrome.

---❖ ❖ ❖---

Jessica is a 48 year old woman who runs an online jewelry business who came to see me because she is always tired. She reports that she isn't snoring (per her husband) and notes she sleeps eight hours each night. Despite this, she is exhausted every day. Her previous doctor had sent her for an overnight sleep study at a major medical center. This evaluation did not detect significant sleep apnea, but did find that Jessica's sleep quality was not optimal.

Based on these results, Jessica began to make some changes in her lifestyle in order to improve her sleep quality. One of these changes was to improve her overall activity level. She acknowledged that she was quite sedentary because of work stress and her busy schedule with her family. The data from her fitness tracker showed that she's been averaging only 4,000 steps per day. We spoke about some strategies to increase Jessica's activity level, such as going for a thirty minute walk around mid-day, taking the stairs instead of the elevator, and establishing a consistent exercise program.

As she made these changes, she used a home sleep monitor (a fitness tracker Jessica wears on her wrist) to monitor how these changes affected the quality of her sleep. Within a couple of weeks, her daily step count was up to an average of about 10,500 steps per day. By tracking the quality of her sleep, Jessica found that her sleep dramatically improved over the ensuing weeks. Jessica also noted that her daytime fatigue was much improved. Increasing her daily activity had made a huge difference for Jessica.

◈ ◈ ◈

Habit 27: Allergy-Proof Yourself and Your Environment

Allergy problems have become much more common in recent years. Allergy issues can include classic types of allergies (itchy eyes, runny nose, hives, etc.) as well as sensitivities (which can manifest as skin reactions or intestinal symptoms). Some of the recommendations in this section may not apply to every type of allergy issue. However, these tools form an "allergy protocol" that will help you combat many of the most common problems.

When I started out in practice in 1995, most patients told me they did not have any allergy problems. However, now about half of the patients I see at UCLA report that they're experiencing an allergy problem in certain situations or certain times of years. If you, or someone you know, experience such problems, it is usually best to consult with an allergist or internist for testing and treatment. In conjunction with medical management, there are five strategies that can help minimize the risk of having problems.

1. Allergy-Proof Your Floor
Carpet is Grand Central Station for dust and other allergy-causing triggers. No matter how well you vacuum your carpets or rugs, significant amounts of dust will continue to make a home there. In addition, every time you vacuum, large amounts of dust will enter the air and can circulate for a significant period of time. If you have allergy problems (especially dust-related nasal/sinus/asthma problems), you should strongly consider removing carpets and rugs from as much of your environment as possible, particularly in your bedroom and other heavily trafficked rooms. After that, be sure to regularly clean floors and shelves to prevent the accumulation of dust.

2. Allergy-Proof Your Bed
Have you ever noticed that many allergy problems happen at night or during sleep? This is because some of the most common allergy exposures are found right in the bedroom. I'm referring to mattresses, pillows, and sheets. Mattresses and pillows, in particular, can be a haven for dust and other exposures so it is important to protect allergy sufferers by using a mattress encasement and pillow encasements. These are specialized barriers that seal the mattress and pillows to reduce the

risk that you will be exposed to allergy triggers during sleep. Encasements have become much easier to find these days and can usually be found at stores such as Target and Wal-Mart or at many online retailers. Sheets and pillowcases can then be used on top of these encasements like you normally would do. It's also important to remember is to wash sheets and pillowcases in hot water once a week. This is important to keep these items clean and as allergy-free as possible.

3. Shower Before Sleep

There is another major reason why sleep is a common time for allergy problems. You may not realize this, but many parts of the environment accumulate on your skin and hair as you go through your day. This includes remnants from trees, grass, dust, and makeup. When you go to bed with this accumulation still on your body, you can transfer these allergens to your sheets and pillowcases. Thus, it can help to shower before bedtime.

4. Consider Eliminating Common Allergy-Inducing Foods

Food allergies are very common. Most of us know people with sensitivities and allergies to certain foods. While many foods and chemicals in the food chain (colorings, preservatives, etc.) can trigger allergy problems, eight foods account for a large percentage of such problems.

1. Wheat
2. Dairy (especially cow's milk)
3. Soy
4. Eggs
5. Tree nuts (cashews, walnuts, almonds, pecans etc.)
6. Peanuts
7. Fish
8. Shellfish

These foods are common causes of allergy problems which can go undiagnosed for years or even decades. Part of the problem is that some of these foods (especially wheat, dairy, and soy) are ubiquitous in the modern food chain. Often, we don't think of food as a possible cause of medical problems. However, these eight foods are common causes of problems ranging from intestinal symptoms to sinus problems to skin problems. Removing all eight of these foods from one's diet is difficult and usually not necessary. However, a sequential elimination diet can be helpful in many cases. To do this, remove one item at a time from your diet to see if symptoms improve. This process should always be practiced under the supervision of a board-certified physician with experience with allergy problems. Keep in mind that each type of food should be removed from your diet for at least three to six months as it can take that long for an improvement to be noted. During this process, be careful to look for these foods in places you might not expect such as supplements, toothpaste, and mouthwash. The elimination diet can help identify any culprits in the food chain that may be contributing to your allergy problems. In general, do your best to avoid foods that contain colorings and other additives as these can also be common causes of food allergies.

5. Air Purification

We all know it's not optimal to breathe cigarette smoke and that second-hand smoke should be avoided. While we accept that cigarette smoke is damaging to our bodies, we often don't consider the health consequences of breathing the air pollution found in so many big cities. In 2007, the prestigious *New England Journal of Medicine* published an article establishing a direct relationship between the level of air pollution in one's community and the risk of dying from heart disease. Other studies have confirmed that your life expectancy is related to how much air pollution you breathe. It's clear that the quality of the air you breathe has a significant effect on health—and that bad air quality is a problem, regardless of what causes the poor air quality.

So, what are we to do? Most books that deal with this topic urge us to advocate for stricter air emissions controls in our local communities. That is definitely important in the long term as improving air quality is the ultimate solution to this problem. In the meantime, I encourage you to focus on what you can do to immediately improve air quality for yourself and for your family. My first recommendation is to place a HEPA air purifier in each bedroom of your house. I prefer the stand-alone individual room HEPA air purifiers because they're mobile and relatively inexpensive. However, installing a total house purification system is another option.

I frequently hear from people that air purifiers aren't important because you need to go outside or spend time in buildings that don't have good air purification systems. Thus, why should people go through the expense of having a bedroom air purifier? My answer to this is that the average person spends about eight hours per day in the bedroom, which is one-third of your life. If you have a high quality air purifier in your bedroom, that means that one-third of the time you're breathing in better quality air. Secondly, many people who work outside the home also spend much of their workday in an office. If those people also put an air purifier in their office space, then nearly two-thirds of their day could be spent in a room with high quality air. The key is to optimize the amount of time that you spend in rooms with good air quality.

What should you look for in an air purifier? First, make sure it does not have an ionizer. Ionizers don't appear to significantly improve air quality and some of them emit ozone which can precipitate asthma problems. Second, measure the room and make sure that the purifier is strong enough to filter the air in a room of that size. Most companies put the room size specifications on the box to make this process easier. Look for the CADR (clean air density rate) for the machine you're considering. This measures how much volume of air the machine can filter per minute. In general, look for CADR's or over 150 for most normal sized rooms. Very large rooms may require higher rates. Third, ensure that the air purifier is a HEPA air purifier. The HEPA specification means that it removes of at least 99.97% of particles from the air that are 0.3 micrometers in size or larger. Fourth, make certain that the machine is from a reputable company that has a proven track record for effectiveness. Finally, please be sure to check the filters regularly and change them per the manufacturer's recommendations or when they look dirty. The filters can be a bit expensive for some of these machines, so check out the replacement filter prices before you buy the unit.

If possible, purchase a HEPA air purifier for your bedroom and/or office space and remember to change the filters when necessary. Also, consider having a HEPA unit in other rooms where you spend more than a few hours per day. While I'm on the subject of indoor air quality, I want to also remind you to be sure to change the filters in your home's furnace on a regular schedule (typically every 2-3 months depending on how often you run your air system).

If you're suffering from allergy issues, make it a priority to practice the strategies discussed in this habit of *The Wellness Code*.

Habit 28: Find Joy

Many of these habits deal with some very serious topics. Well, this not one of them. This is the fun habit of incorporating joy into your life. Did you know that laughing, smiling, and having fun are actually good for your health? It turns out that happiness is truly good for you, which is why joy is a key component of *The Wellness Code*.

A recent study from The University of Maryland Medical Center found that laughing was associated with a lower rate of heart disease. Another study found that laughter reduced measures of inflammation within the body and even improved cholesterol levels. Yet another study showed that laughter improved the health of diabetic patients. There is compelling evidence that laughter, smiling, and having fun are truly beneficial to your health in many different ways.

Many serious, "Type A" people often forget how important it is to laugh, smile, and have fun. Science is starting to catch up on this as studies are now showing the clear connection between happiness and health. Smiling, laughing and having fun are actually good for your health. Make sure that smiling and laughing are a regular part of your daily life.

One important lesson in this regard is that it's more important to find joy in your everyday life than it is to plan activities in an effort to find happiness. This is a very important concept to accept and bring into your life. Find a way to add humor and laughter to your ordinary day rather than only having fun on weekends or during your vacation. If you have children, you know that adding humor and happiness to your everyday interactions will make parenting your children easier and much more pleasant. Happiness should flow naturally from what you do every day.

Sometimes this isn't easy as bad things happen and life can be difficult at times. However, finding joy is most important during stressful times. Regardless of what is going on, try to find at least a few minutes to find something that brings you pleasure. It can be watching a television sitcom, listening to great music, going to a party, or just hearing a good joke. Be proactive and find ways to make life fun and enjoyable.

Think of some creative ways to practice this habit. Don't let negative forces in the world dictate your mood. Create opportunities to smile. It turns out that a smile is contagious. When you smile, others will smile. A laugh or a smile can be passed through a home or an office just like a memo. Be sure to laugh and smile every single day. It's a fun thing to do and it promotes wellness.

Habit 29: Practice Hobbies

Finding time for a hobby has become a challenge in recent years. It's easy to get consumed with work and family life, but it is important to maintain your personal interests. Specifically, it's important to your health to have hobbies unrelated to your work or home life. Participating in meaningful hobbies has been linked to a reduced risk of stroke, heart attack, and memory loss.

Do you currently have hobbies that you enjoy on a regular basis? If not, think back to your younger days. What hobbies did you enjoy before life got so busy? Was it a musical instrument? Was it a sport? Was it reading? Was it something else? What were the activities that you would joyfully practice even if you didn't have to do so? Which activities did you find yourself doing when you had nothing else scheduled? Think of activities where you found meaning and true inspiration. These were the hobbies that you thought about night and day.

Having a hobby is important because doing something purely because it makes you happy and fulfilled is a way for you to stay connected to yourself and sometimes to a higher calling. Most of the time, the majority of waking hours involves connecting with others and meeting needs outside of yourself. That's why hobbies are so very important. Hobbies allow you to find deeper meaning so you will be better able to meet your external obligations. As the safety instructions on an airplane say, "Put on your own oxygen mask before assisting others."

Outside of my main career, I have a lot of hobbies including listening to music, running, writing, and creating podcasts. When I think of these hobbies, I get really motivated and excited. Which hobbies have the same effect on you? Think back to your childhood. Which were the activities that your parents didn't need to force you to do? Try to find at least one or two activities that you can enjoy each week. It should ideally be something about which you're passionate. It should also be something that can conveniently fit into your schedule each week. For example, you may love golf, but simply don't have the time to play golf each week, so golf may not be the ideal hobby for you.

Notice that I didn't say that you need to be skilled at this activity— you just need to enjoy it. You need to savor it. You may be an awful piano player, but it may still be a wonderful hobby for you if you enjoy playing this instrument and find great inspiration in it. Once you've picked your hobbies of choice, set aside time for them each week. Hobbies can have a powerful effect on your health and well-being. Be sure to make this a regular part of your life.

◈ ◈ ◈

Barry is a 68 year old vice president of a Fortune 500 company. He came to see me the month before he retired because he wanted to have a health assessment before embarking on the next stage of his life. He was on multiple medications for high blood pressure, diabetes, and high cholesterol. Despite these medications, his cholesterol and sugars levels were both elevated and his blood pressure readings were not well-controlled. He told me that he has never practiced a healthy lifestyle and that he has spent the last forty years working long hours and largely ignoring his health. We then reviewed his nutrition and exercise habits and we agreed on a plan for him to improve those areas going forward.

I asked Barry if he had a plan for his retirement and told me that he was feeling a bit nervous as he wasn't sure what he would be doing on a day-to-day basis. He was married and was excited to spend more time with his wife. He was also looking forward to spending more time with his adult children and his grandchildren. I asked Barry if he had a hobby from childhood or young adulthood that he might return to in the coming months. He smiled and told me about his love of the bass guitar. He played all through childhood and was even in a band in his 20's. He then mentioned his love of golf, which he used to play in his younger days. All of a sudden, Barry straightened up and said he was excited to get back to these hobbies that he used to love so much. I joked that he might consider playing bass guitar in a band that performs at golf tournaments and he smiled in a way that let me know that his transition into retirement would be a smooth one. Barry returned to see me later that year and I was amazed at how much healthier he looked. Now retired, he was playing golf several times a week and also taking bass guitar lessons. I was amazed to see how active he had become. I was also thrilled to see how well-controlled his blood pressure, diabetes, and cholesterol levels were. This was likely as a result of his improved activity level and his reduced stress level.

$$\diamond \; \diamond \; \diamond$$

Set aside an hour or two a week to practice a hobby that brings you pleasure. Table 3, at the end of this book, provides a list of possible hobbies if you're looking to explore new possibilities. If you aren't sure what you want to do, think back to your life when you had fewer obligations and more free time. What did you enjoy doing then? Once you have your answer, make time for it on your calendar.

Habit 30: Simplify Your Life

Have you ever thought about what makes a vacation a relaxing experience? I've found that one of the nicest aspects of being on vacation is that the hotel room is clean and uncluttered. In contrast to most homes, a hotel room isn't filled with things you need to clean, fix, put away or file. In addition, your schedule on vacation is usually pretty relaxed and open-ended. I find that it is the very absence of physical and mental clutter that contributes to the rejuvenating effect of going on vacation.

Of course, it's usually not possible to live your daily life with an open-ended schedule and as few possessions as on vacation. However, by simplifying your life, you will be able to reduce stress and make your day-to-day life more vacation-like. It's a good rule of thumb that, if you find yourself nearly paralyzed by the sheer volume of your commitments and your possessions, then your life would likely benefit from simplification.

Physical Clutter

Physical clutter makes it difficult to focus your attention and truly enjoy yourself in the moment. Why? If something is in your visual space, it creates a distraction which inevitably leads to a new thought pattern. This is why studying at a library is often more productive than at home. Fewer distractions mean easier concentration. It is difficult to stay engaged in what you are doing when your attention is constantly being diverted by something else. Perhaps you're lying on the couch reading a mystery novel and trying to stay engrossed in the story. However, nearby are stacks of papers you need to file, mail that needs to be opened, and dishes that need to be rinsed. Every time your eyes drift from your book, you see one of these items and suddenly your thoughts become worries about all of the chores you need to do. This makes it very difficult to be fully embrace relaxation and truly enjoy your book.

Many of us love to keep things. I'm one of those people. Throwing things out is simply not in my nature, so I need to work extra hard on the habit of simplifying and de-cluttering. If you wake up one day and realize that every corner of your home is being used to store all of your stuff from years ago, it's time to remove some of the clutter. You know what I mean: your notebooks from high school, receipts from 1995, and your driver's license from 1992. Perhaps that's just me?

A lot of us hold on to things because we think we might need to use them again in the future. This isn't a big deal when you only have two or three boxes of stuff, but slowly over time you build up a collection of dozens of boxes filling up your closets and your storage areas. Then you have a big problem. Even if there were things in those boxes that you may want to use, you would probably never be able to find them. Recently, I spent hours looking for an important book—sorting through countless boxes of books I have never read and probably never will—hoping that each box would have that particular book inside. All this clutter means that important things aren't readily accessible when you need them.

Also, while these items sit gathering dust in your attic, basement, and closets, there are people in your community who would benefit greatly from each of these items. This is one of the reasons there are so many charities out there that can help find a home for that book sitting in your attic or that sofa in your basement. There's a family out there who could really use that couch or Halloween costume from so many years ago. Holding on to all that stuff means that other people are missing out on using these items.

Also, I would argue that keeping so many old items wears on you spiritually. There is something liberating about letting go of the things you don't need any longer to keep your life as simple as possible. Letting go of what you don't need allows you to enjoy what's truly important in life.

Try keeping only what you need and use. When you hold on to old items that don't have a purpose in your life, you're metaphorically holding on to your past experiences in a way that detracts from your present. There's a liberating freedom to letting go of your past and starting fresh each day unencumbered and free. We will return to this concept in future habits such as habit 42 and habit 50.

Make it a habit to simplify and streamline your physical possessions. Possibly needing something in the future isn't always a good reason to keep something. A good rule of thumb is to donate or sell anything that you haven't used in the past three years. If you are drowning in clutter, it can be difficult to know where to start. I recommend starting with these baby steps.

1. Paperwork

Go through all the papers that you've accumulated over the years. Set aside a box for the papers that you need to keep and recycle the rest. To avoid identity theft, shred any paperwork that has personal information such as a social security number, account numbers, or personal financial information. I recommend dealing with your paperwork one pile or one box at a time. Some find it easier to spend an hour per day on this. Others prefer to sort through all of their old paperwork in a weekend. Try whatever is most comfortable for you. Once you are caught up, be sure to have a system in place to keep up with new paperwork. Create a filing system so you won't have to deal with a mountain of paperwork ever again. Consider scanning paperwork and archiving the electronic copies using an online cloud storage system such as Dropbox, Google Drive, or Copy.com. Many people take photos of their children's artwork and create a photobook using Shutterfly or VistaPrint.

Getting a handle on the paperwork in your life will ensure that bills get paid on time, paperwork is readily accessible when you need it, and you no longer have to move piles of paper when you want to have people over to your house. The end result of all of that is a reduction in stress and more time to enjoy your life.

2. Physical items:

Before you sort through your possessions, start by creating designated areas to help you sort and dispose of the items that are cluttering your living space. It is much easier to get a handle on the physical items if you have a place to put them. I recommend labeling three boxes as follows: keep, trash, and donate. To get started, pick out the areas that bother you the most because of physical clutter. For many people, this would mean their kitchen or bedroom.

Unless you have lots of free time and a burning desire to sort through your possessions, I recommend starting with one portion of a room at a time. For a bedroom, this could mean that you start by just decluttering your bedside table. In a kitchen, you could sort through cookbooks so you only keep the ones you use. As you pare down each category and maintain the order and usefulness of that area, you will likely be inspired to address additional areas as time permits. And, day-by-day, your habit of getting rid of the items that aren't benefitting your life will slowly result in a more orderly and peaceful home.

Mental Clutter

In addition to removing physical clutter from your life, it's important to also remove clutter from your mind. Take a step back and think through what you did with your time over the past week. How much time did you spend connecting in a positive way with your friends, family and community? How much time did you spend doing something that gives you pleasure, such as practicing a hobby (habit 29)? It's important to ensure that the majority of your waking hours are spent doing work you find fulfilling. It's also important to spend time with people who add positivity to your life. Reducing mental clutter is a prerequisite for making this happen.

One important step in reducing your mental clutter is to evaluate your relationships and take active steps to nurture the relationships that help you be a more positive person. Think about whether you're spending time with people who focus on gossip and negativity. Life is too short to maintain relationships with people who drag you down instead of lift you up. Reach out to the people with whom you enjoy spending time and schedule time with them.

Streamline your schedule so that the majority of your time is spent doing things you find meaningful. Doing so will promote an environment that helps to keep stress levels at bay. While it is good to have all of the important parts of life scheduled into your calendar, be sure to have some free time available for spontaneous experiences. When your schedule is over-packed, all the "stuff" in your life can become overwhelming and create tremendous stress that can actually detract from your wellness. At that point, your schedule goes from being "interesting and fulfilling" to "taxing and overwhelming." Often you don't realize when this transition occurs as it usually happens gradually over time. Make sure that most of your scheduled events enrich your life or someone else's life in some way. Habit 21 detailed how to plan your calendar. Review your schedule on a regular basis and start saying "no" to things that add excessive stress to your life and prioritize those that add meaning. Simplify the clutter in your calendar on a regular basis.

◆ ◆ ◆

Linda is a 38 year old patient with a history of rheumatoid arthritis (RA) who came to see me because she was having increasing trouble getting around her house. She was on multiple medications which helped a bit, but the pain in her knees, hips, and hands had become quite severe.

Linda told me she managed her pain by working out at the gym five days a week, attending a meditation class three days a week, going to a support group twice a week, meeting with her physical therapist twice a week, seeing a chiropractor once a week, and the list went on and on.

Linda seemed exhausted just describing her busy schedule. Linda also confided that she's only getting five hours of sleep a night and her job performance at work has slipped. Her intentions were in the right place as she was trying to do everything that could possibly help her condition. However, she was running herself into the ground by overcommitting herself and this was affecting her health.

I worked with Linda to prioritize her schedule and focus on the activities that were giving her the most benefit. I told her that getting a good night sleep is paramount and it wasn't possible to participate in all of these activities and still get sufficient quality sleep. Moreover, her schedule was adding stress to her life, which we know is detrimental to patients with autoimmune diseases like rheumatoid arthritis. Overextending herself in an effort to try every possible treatment may be actually hurting her chances for a recovery.

We also discussed that she was forgetting to take her medications because the dosing schedule of her pills was very complicated. Thus, I adjusted some of her prescription medications to simplify the dosing schedule.

She returned to see me one month later feeling like a new person. She looked like she had just returned from a vacation feeling refreshed and alive. Her stress level was much improved and she was sleeping much better with her treatment regimen streamlined and simplified.

◈ ◈ ◈

Go through your home, your office, your car, and your schedule on a regular basis and get rid of whatever excess "baggage" you've been carrying. Simplify your life. Remember that less can be more.

Habit 31: Take a Break

Life can be overwhelmingly busy at times. Sometimes it seems like there are fewer hours in the day. The truth is the length of the day hasn't changed, but how much we want to accomplish in those hours has risen dramatically.

Smartphones and other technological advances were supposed to lead to more free time, but the opposite has turned out to be the case. We are now all instantaneously available and have unlimited information at our fingertips, which means that the workday never ends for many people. Even during leisure time, maintaining and mastering a variety of electronic devices eats into our already time-constrained lives.

Sometimes it seems like just keeping all of your devices charged is a full-time job. In the midst of this constant availability and connectedness, it is so easy to forget the importance of recharging yourself. For your physical and mental health, you need to recharge your internal batteries on a regular basis and this works best when the recharging happens one full day per week.

If you don't take the time to recharge your body and soul, you will burn out.

In an ideal world, you would give up TV, computers, and even your electronic devices for one day each week. Use this "unplugged" day to reconnect with friends and family. You can enjoy a relaxing meal together. You might even read a good book and snooze on the couch. There's so much you can do to recharge yourself that doesn't involve technology and doing more work. The key is to turn off your busy work life, whether it's at the office or at home, and take time to explore the areas of life that tend to be forgotten all week.

For some, it's impossible to completely turn off technology for one full day, so I suggest starting slowly. Perhaps try not using technology for one evening each week. The thought of doing so may seem unrealistic, but your soul needs this time, and your wellness depends on it.

◆ ◆ ◆

Carlos is a 46 years old sports executive who came to me because he felt burnt out. He's been working extremely long hours and has been traveling on business trips every other week for the past year. He said his energy level was down and his nutrition and exercise habits had been less than ideal for quite a while. Carlos said he felt that the way he was living his life was out of touch with his core values.

I asked him what he considered to be his core values and he said he values three things: friends, family, and his faith. However, he also said that providing for his family is a priority, but that he has taken this to an extreme level recently. He told me that his marriage is on shaky ground and he doesn't feel connected to his kids anymore.

Carlos and I spoke for a long time and he told me that his weekday schedule is simply jam-packed. He leaves the house at 6 am and typically gets home at 8 or 9 pm. I asked him about his weekends and he said that Sundays are a bit lighter for him. I proposed that he designate Sunday as his friends and family day: his day of rest and connection. I explained that he needed time each week to rest, rejuvenate, and connect with those closest to him. He looked interested, but questioned if he could set aside a full day each week. I asked him to begin by setting aside every Sunday morning until noon to spend time with friends and family away from work. Carlos promised that every Sunday morning would be his time to focus on his priorities—his family, his friends, and his faith. A few weeks later, I received an email from Carlos' son thanking me for helping to bring his dad back.

◆ ◆ ◆

Take one day each week and focus on connecting with friends and family. Don't go on the Internet. Don't watch TV. Don't deal with work. Try it out. You'll be amazed how much better and more productive you are the rest of the workweek. Give it a shot and you will likely start to look forward to this each week. The time away from the online world is refreshing and rejuvenating. Try this for a week or two and I promise you'll be hooked.

Habit 32: Read Every Day

Reading is also a part of *The Wellness Code*. Specifically, make it a goal to read a book unrelated to your profession or home life for thirty minutes each day. Reading is important because it stimulates the brain by feeding your creativity and imagination. Reading is in some ways a lost art, but has vital effects on your mind and your overall wellness. In particular, reading something outside of your profession or home-related issues is important to your personal growth. It takes you out of the flow of regular life and can serve as a sort of daily vacation for the mind.

Think about what sorts of things you might read during your thirty minutes. You could use this time to read about a hobby (habit 29) which could be history, sports, music, movies, fashion, cars, or any other topic that interests you. Your reading choice could be fiction or nonfiction. Fiction feeds your creative juices while nonfiction feeds your thirst for knowledge. The key is to make reading a daily habit. The goal is to redirect your mind away from work and family matters for at least thirty minutes each day. Try it out. Spend some time putting together a reading list. If you are having trouble coming up with books that appeal to you, check out online book retailers, local bookstores, or your library. Another good way to get book recommendations is to use Facebook to ask friends to share their current favorite books. Make sure that these are books that you *want* to read, not that you think you *should* read. These may be books that you've wanted to read for years. Now's the time. Get started today.

◈ ◈ ◈

Peter is a 53 year old contractor who came to see me as a new patient because of recently diagnosed type 2 diabetes. Peter and I discussed his new diagnosis and reviewed all the basics of proper nutrition, exercise, and sleep management. I prescribed medication to help regulate his blood sugar levels. Peter also needed to lose some weight and he confessed that he was consuming far too much bread, sweets, and pasta. Peter said his biggest struggle was to avoid snacking on sugar-rich foods at night as he usually sits in front of the television and snacks on cookies and chips while he watches ESPN.

We spoke about some strategies like removing unhealthy snacks from his home and replacing them with healthy snacks. We also discussed strategies to help break his habit of snacking in front of the television. Peter told me that he used to be an avid reader and would love to get back into reading. We brainstormed for a few minutes and discussed reading books about sports including fiction and nonfiction options. We agreed this was a good idea because reading focuses the mind and the attention in much healthier ways than television. In Peter's case, he started to read books about exercise and also about some of his favorite athletes. Reading those books inspired him to start exercising and he joined a local gym. Before long, he was working out five times per week and his sugar levels improved. This was a terrific first step as Peter was beginning to break his old habits and replace them with habits that promote a healthier lifestyle.

◆ ◆ ◆

In my family, we schedule reading at the end of each day, just before going to bed. This provides numerous benefits in that reading helps improve sleep habits (habit 26) and also improves memory and concentration. After we instituted this rule for our children, we quickly noticed significant improvements at school and in their overall focus. I've been amazed how it calms our children and helps them relax after a long day at school or playing sports. Reading is also incredibly helpful for adults as well. Make reading a part of your daily routine and you will see many benefits.

Habit 33: Volunteer Each Week

Volunteering is a habit that provides you with an incredible return on your investment. In addition to giving back to your community, volunteering your time actually improves your health. One study from The University of Michigan found that patients who volunteer each week live longer and have improved risk factors for heart disease and stroke. Research suggests that volunteering for just two hours per week or about 100 hours per year is enough to provide significant health benefits. Volunteering can be an amazing antidote to the stress and wear and tear of life.

Your volunteer work can be for any worthwhile cause or organization such as a school, a place of worship, or something related to a hobby of yours. For most, it is best to volunteer in an area where you have some expertise or passion. Thus, if you play piano, perhaps you could offer free piano lessons to disadvantaged children. If you're a soccer player, perhaps you could become a volunteer soccer coach or give soccer lessons. If you're a health professional, perhaps you could volunteer in neighborhoods without access to health services. The key is to donate your time and effort with no expectation of anything in return.

Think about how you might expand your volunteer time each week and each year. There's something powerful about stepping outside of yourself and focusing on others who are in need.

❖ ❖ ❖

Kim is 36 year old patient of mine who came to see me after her dentist found that her blood pressure was elevated. We discussed the significance of her elevated blood pressure readings and the lifestyle issues that were likely impacting these numbers. We focused on sleep, stress, exercise, and diet. Because her blood pressure readings were extremely elevated, I prescribed a medication to lower her blood pressure. As part of our discussion about stress, Kim mentioned a particular issue she's been having with her 11 year old daughter Sophia. Sophia was not showing much consideration for others, either at home or at school. I could see Kim's stress level begin to rise as she spoke about her daughter. She said it was incredibly painful to see her daughter becoming so self-centered with so little regard for others. I suggested that Kim find ways for the two of them to get involved with a charity organization where they could volunteer together. We discussed that one of the best ways to help a child become less self-involved is to get her involved in activities that help others. I also asked Kim to return in a month to reevaluate her blood pressure.

At Kim's return visit, her blood pressure reading was close to normal. Kim said her stress was much improved because her relationship with her daughter was much better. Kim had found a local nursing home where children and their parents can volunteer. Once each week, Sophia and Kim spent the afternoon at the home helping the elderly residents. Kim said that she had noticed a dramatic shift in her daughter's attitude. Sophia was starting to show more consideration for other people and her demeanor was becoming much more upbeat and less sullen. Volunteering was helping Sophia, but Kim's stress level was also much improved as well.

❖ ❖ ❖

When you plan your weekly schedule, be sure to include about two hours of volunteer work. Find a place where you can lend your time and/or expertise to help someone or some group of people. Volunteer ideas are listed in table 4 at the end of this book. By volunteering, you'll be helping others and helping yourself.

Habit 34: Love Your Self

There's no doubt that relationships have a significant impact on your health and longevity. This habit of *The Wellness Code* focuses on one of your most important relationships, which is your relationship with yourself.

Your relationship with yourself is crucial to your health and well-being. We've all heard about self-worth, self-love, or similar concepts. Self-love does not mean that you are a self-centered, narcissistic person. It does not mean that you like everything about yourself. For example, there may be something about your personality that you may not like. Perhaps you are quick to become jealous or angry; self-love does not mean that you love these aspects of your personality, just that you accept that they are a part of who you are at this time.

Self-love is comprised of four main components.

The first step of self-love is observation. You observe yourself and you see yourself for who you really are at the current time. For example, if you have a jealous streak, recognize that instead of denying that it exists. Look at your characteristics honestly, try your best to understand them and work with them. Observe yourself and be honest with yourself about who you really are—the good and the bad. Observing yourself is important, but be careful not to turn this into self-blame and self-hatred. That's how self-worth gets degraded and falls apart. While you see yourself for who you are right now, you also envision the kind of the person that you hope to become down the road.

The second step of self-love is kindness. When you see a blind man struggling to walk down the street, you reach out your hand and help him across the busy intersection. When your newborn baby continues to cry because she has a fever, you hold and soothe her. It's important to show yourself the same sort of kindness and compassion that you show others in need. Try to be patient with yourself and show yourself some kindness. We all sometimes struggle; remember that when you're having trouble with some aspect of life.

The third step of self-love is acceptance. By acceptance I do not mean that you accept that a negative trait should continue to be a part of your personality. Rather, you accept that this is your reality right now. If you get jealous easily, it doesn't serve any purpose to get angry about it or hate yourself. Rather, accept that this is the reality of how things are right now. In some ways this may seem counterintuitive, but once you accept that something is true about yourself, you will be positioning yourself to begin to change that aspect of yourself and grow as a person. It is only when you see yourself for who you are and fully embrace and accept that truth, can you grow as a person.

This leads to step four of self-love: attention. After observation, kindness, and acceptance, it's important to give your attention to those aspects of yourself that need the most attention. Perhaps you have a tendency to close off and become isolated during times of stress. Perhaps you have a tendency to procrastinate. Focus on the skills you need to strengthen in both your personal and professional lives. Be sure to remember to circle back to the prior steps and continue to observe yourself, give yourself kindness, practice acceptance, and pay the necessary attention to grow as a person.

This is so important because you can't have a healthy relationship with others without first having a healthy relationship with yourself. Having a healthy relationship with yourself is a pivotal building block in *The Wellness Code*.

Make it a practice to keep a personal journal. Use this as a tool to focus on your relationship with yourself. Use each entry to evaluate how you handled a situation, and whether you are pleased with how you handled it. For example, if you realized that you expressed your irritation with a colleague in a less than constructive way, use this as an opportunity to think through the incident and re-evaluate the interaction so that you'll do better next time. Apply the concepts of observation, kindness, acceptance, and attention so you can understand why you handled things in a way you regret and can make a plan to do things differently in the future.

This exercise will help you expand on the positive aspects of your personality and give attention to the areas on which you'd like to improve. If you practice this, you will become a more compassionate person—both to yourself and to others—which will result in less stress and better health. By growing your self-worth and self-awareness, you will put yourself in a position to have rewarding relationships with others, which will be the topic for subsequent habits.

Habit 35: Love Your Spouse or Partner

In habit 34, I discussed the importance of self-worth as a precursor to being able to sustain healthy relationships with others. Studies have consistently shown that healthy relationships directly impact both the quality of your health and your longevity. Your relationships have emotional, cognitive, physical, and spiritual effects on your wellness.

One of the most important relationships is with your spouse or partner. If you have grown in your self-worth and developed your relationship skills, then you are poised to make your primary intimate relationship thrive. There are many studies showing that having a healthy, intimate, monogamous relationship promotes good health.

When I say intimate relationship, I'm referring to more than just physical intimacy. I'm also referring to true, deep emotional love. The two main components of a healthy, intimate monogamous relationship are a physical and an emotional connection.

The first component is the physical component. There is a power to physical connection through touch. Human beings are meant to experience touch and that physical connection is crucial in promoting good health. For an intimate relationship to flourish, intimate relations need to be a priority. However, physical intimacy should ideally include many different forms of physical connection, not just sexual relations. This means holding hands. It means holding each other in bed. It means sharing a kiss each morning. The key is to maintain a level of physical intimacy and physical contact on a consistent basis.

The second component of true intimacy goes beyond just a physical connection and involves the emotional side of your relationship. Some couples spend a lifetime together and yet never share their deepest thoughts and feelings. To be truly intimate with your spouse or partner, you need to be able and willing to be honest—completely honest and emotionally vulnerable.

Robin is a 52 year old patient who has been experiencing significant sleep problems which have become more severe in recent months. She finds herself waking during the night for no apparent reason. Recently, she was so tired that she fell asleep while driving and crashed into a stop sign. She suffered severe injuries to her left shoulder, which ultimately required surgery. Her husband convinced her to see me to see if we could improve her sleep patterns. There was no history of snoring and no apparent reason for her sleep issues. I took a careful history looking for any possible reason for her sleep problems. Robin told me that work was going well and that the last of their three kids had just left for college and that they were a source of joy to her. I then asked about her marriage and commented to Robin that some marital strains become apparent when the couple becomes empty nesters.

Robin mentioned that she and her husband had been struggling for years, but lately things had gotten a lot worse. Robin said that they haven't been emotionally close for several years, ever since the death of her husband's parents. Robin said that he was deeply affected by their death and since then he hasn't communicated well with her. She told me that the intimacy in their marriage vanished. When the kids were at home, it wasn't so bad, but now that they are all off to college, the emotional void in their relationship had become difficult to handle. Robin told me that the toughest thing for her has been the lack of emotional and physical connection. As Robin's sleep issues were likely related to this stress, I recommended that she ask her husband if he might consider marital counseling and gave her the names of several excellent local therapists. Several months later, I received a phone call from Robin that she and her husband were in couple's therapy and things had improved. In particular, her sleep habits were just about back to normal, and her recovery from her shoulder surgery was going well.

❖ ❖ ❖

It is extremely important to prioritize your relationship with your spouse or partner. Nurture your relationship and take care of it on a daily basis so that it grows over time and doesn't fade away. Schedule "dates" to make sure you spend quality time together on a regular basis.

Ideas for "date nights" are listed in table 5 at the end of this book. If you don't have common interests, find one. Every couple has a common interest if you look hard enough. Listen to each other and try to see things from the others' perspective. Make this a priority. Moreover, if you're currently married or involved in a monogamous relationship, make sure that you are intimate each day—this doesn't necessarily mean that you're having sex every day, but be sure to maintain the emotional connection on a daily basis. You need to find time to have deep conversations and free-spirited fun times as well.

Just as you spend time investing in your retirement account, invest in your primary intimate relationship. Don't take this precious relationship for granted. Those that take it for granted tend to be the ones who are eventually looking for a new relationship later in life. The stress of a broken intimate relationship can have profound effects on wellness. Stay proactive and be engaged in your relationship with your spouse or partner. It's vitally important to a long and healthy life.

Habit 36: Love Your Children

This habit addresses how one of the most important jobs that you will ever have—parenting— has a profound effect on wellness. Specifically, how you parent will affect the health of your children in countless ways. Many studies have shown that high quality parenting improves the chances that your children will practice healthy habits in regard to nutrition and exercise. Moreover, effective parenting promotes a low stress environment which is conducive to good health.

You may be thinking that you aren't a parent, or you may have no plans to be a parent. This habit still applies because just about every single person will have some kind of parental role in their lifetime. Perhaps you'll play this role for a niece, nephew, or friend. We all have an impact on the younger generation who will one day grow up to be adults. The impact you have on children has exponential effects on the world. This is because children will interact with so many other people in their lives. Thus, the impact that you have on one child can have a far-reaching impact on the world. To improve the likelihood that your parenting leads to good consequences, this habit is about practicing effective, positive parenting.

How do you practice effective parenting? Parenting books usually spend chapter after chapter teaching tools for how to deal with tantrums, ADHD symptoms, and every possible challenging behavior. These books discuss what to say to rectify every behavioral issue that can arise. While these techniques can be helpful, the truth is that children learn little from what we say. Scary, right? Children don't learn that much when you tell them to do their homework, get along with their siblings, or say thank you. Those things can help, but not as much as we hope.

Here is what I believe to be the single most important lesson about parenting.

Children learn from what you do, not from what you say.

Children are always watching how you react, how you treat people, what you say, and what you don't say. They learn how you deal with the good and the bad. They learn how you deal with seemingly minor events and major life challenges. They learn all of this by observing you.

If you want to be a really great parent, model the behaviors you want your children to exhibit.

If you want children to say thank you and show kindness to others, make sure that they see you behaving that way on a daily basis. If you want your children to eat healthy foods, then make sure that they see you making good nutritional choices. If you don't want your kids to curse, then make sure that you don't curse. If you want your kids to be kind to others, then show them consistent acts of kindness. For example, let's say you're with your children one morning and you stop by your local coffee shop to get yourself a cup of coffee or tea for yourself. Make it a habit to buy a cup of coffee for a stranger behind you on line. Your children will remember your spontaneous act of kindness and carry that message with them.

Children may not seem to be paying attention, but, trust me, they're watching you. They're learning how to deal with situations by watching you. They're learning what makes a healthy adult relationship by watching how the adults around them get along or don't get along. These are the relationship models that they have. They keep the memories of these relationships in their minds as they grow up and begin to have relationships of their own. They will likely find themselves with friendships like the ones they saw growing up. They will likely find themselves in love relationships like the ones they saw growing up.

Worry less about what you tell your children and focus more on being the kind of person you want them to become. While there is some important value in what you tell your children, how you act in their presence has the most impact on how they develop and who they will be when they grow up.

It's also important to remember to be kind to yourself when you're not the perfect parent. Be compassionate to yourself and do better the next time. Children learn from how we behave, but they also learn from how we respond to adversity. They see us accepting responsibility and striving to improve ourselves and that is an important lesson that they will internalize.

A helpful way to look at what it takes to be a good parent is to consider this definition of a good parent. A good parent is one who only passes on half of his or her "issues" to their children. Do your best to recognize your positive and negative qualities and strive to pass on your positive qualities to your children. Also, make it your goal to reduce the negative qualities that get passed on to the next generation by about fifty percent.

What other factors are most important in practicing effective parenting? The first is having dinner together every night. Studies have shown that one of the best predictors of whether a child will develop good character is whether the family has dinner together most nights. There's something powerful about a family sharing dinner together each night. This is a great opportunity to discuss the events of the day and to discuss challenges as well as accomplishments. Having the chance to discuss things as a family and brainstorm ideas fosters both maturity and growth. The second parenting strategy is for each child to have special time with each parent every week. This doesn't have to be a full day together. It can be a brief walk in the neighborhood. Each child should spend one-on-one time with each parent every week. Just like the family dinner, one-on-one time allows for conversations about important topics and this is crucial in promoting maturity and development.

There are many other important strategies for effective parenting, but I always return to modeling as being most important. Model the kind of behavior that you want your children to learn. Remember that how you behave in front of your children is the single most important parenting strategy there is. Be the kind of person you want your children to become. They're watching you.

Habit 37: Love Your Friends & Family

As I have discussed in several prior habits, staying connected to the important relationships in your life contributes to your health and well-being. Habit 34 discussed the importance of caring for yourself, while habit 35 focused on your relationship with your spouse or partner. Habit 36 was about your relationship to the next generation. Habit 37 focuses on the importance of having strong connections to your friends and family.

You need human connection not just because those connections make you feel better, but because your health literally depends on it. People with few social connections are much more likely to suffer many different types of health problems including heart disease, cancer, and autoimmune disease. These connections can be with a group of friends that gets together for dinner every month, a monthly poker group, or it could be a church or other religious group that meets on a regular basis. The key is to be a part of a community that encourages healthy and supportive relationships. Face-to-face community interactions are usually the best. No matter how much you use social media platforms like Facebook, Twitter, Pinterest, or Instagram, direct human connection is still optimal.

An Australian study showed the importance of human connections by finding that those with close social connection had a 22% reduced risk of death over a ten year period. Another study from Harvard showed that those with close social ties were less likely to have memory problems. There are literally dozens of published studies that have highlighted the benefits of close connections to friends and family.

Another benefit from having a strong social network is that it eases the pressure on your spouse or partner. You and your partner need to have friends and family who you can count on for social and emotional support during the good times as well as the bad times.

--------◈ ◈ ◈--------

Paulina is a 55 year old patient of mine with Crohn's disease who was having increasing diarrhea, bloating, and gas. She was recently seen by her gastroenterologist, who increased some of her medications. She reported feeling a bit better but not truly well. Paulina said that she was coming to me to see if I could suggest anything to help alleviate her worsening intestinal symptoms.

We discussed how problems like Crohn's disease can be aggravated by stress. I asked if she had been experiencing any stress lately, and she said that the past few months had been difficult for her. Her son has been going through a challenging time with his divorce. Paulina is the matriarch of her family and it has been stressful for her to see her son go through such a difficult experience. The more we spoke, the more it became clear that there was a correlation between this stressful experience and the recent problems with her health. I explained to Paulina that this stress was likely contributing to her recent flare-ups. She said that she hasn't spoken with her son in a few weeks, as she didn't know what to say to help him. I suggested she call her son and meet with him regularly. I suggested that she try to just listen and refrain from giving advice or feeling like she needed to fix his situation. I asked her to just be there for him without judgment and without an agenda. Later that week, Paulina had lunch with her son and she simply listened for the entire meal. This was a major step for her. Paulina called me to let me know about her accomplishment and she also told me that she noticed fewer problems with her bowels that week. It was only a first step for Paulina, but it was a very important step indeed.

◈ ◈ ◈

We are social beings and need social connections to other people. Many of us get busy with our work or family lives and don't pay sufficient attention to our friendships and our family relationships. This can result in losing touch with friends and with relatives who we used to see all of the time. Maintaining friendships and close social connections has clear health benefits. It's good for your health and the health of those around you.

Make it a goal to call or visit at least one friend or family member each week. Make this a part of your weekly schedule.

Habit 38: Participate in Your Community

Just as it is critical to stay connected to your spouse or partner, children, friends, and family, it is also essential to stay connected to your community. By community, I mean your local, national, and even international community. It's become a bit of a cliché to say this, but our world has expanded over the past couple of generations to the point where we are all interconnected. With the advent of the Internet, our circles of contact have grown immeasurably. It used to be more difficult to maintain close contacts outside of your own town or city, but that has changed thanks to technological advances.

What does this mean in regard to your health, longevity, and happiness? Well, staying connected to your community is clearly vital to your wellness. Those who feel isolated and alone have a much greater risk of almost every possible medical problem. Let me repeat that.

Those who feel isolated and alone have a much greater risk of almost every medical problem.

The challenge that we face is that it has actually become much more difficult to stay connected to your community even with all the social media platforms at our disposal. It used to be that you could stay connected by simply going to the grocery store, the post office, or local town events. All the people you wanted to see were at those places, and catching up and staying in touch wasn't so challenging.

Well, it's not so easy anymore. While social media have made superficial contact much easier, it has actually become more difficult to have truly significant and deeply rooted interactions. Many people pride themselves on having hundreds or thousands of "friends" when they may only truly connect with a few of those people on a real emotional level.

The solution to this dilemma is to focus on meaningful connections in your life. Having tons of friends on social media looks nice, but consider what really adds meaning to your life. Social media may have a role in your world, but using these sites as a substitute for true human interaction can actually be detrimental to your health. Receiving scores of "likes" for a status update simply doesn't provide the same level of benefit for your wellness as actually interacting with members of your community on a face-to-face basis.

The key to connecting with your community is to find opportunities where deep human connection is fostered. One of the easiest ways to help stay connected to your community is to attend regular events with a secular or religious organization. Find an organization that shares your values and then plan regular time with this community. There are many different types of organizations that can fill this need. Examples include most houses of worship, PTSAs, Habitat for Humanity, or any of thousands of other wonderful organizations. The key is to find a group of people with whom you find a significant and meaningful connection and find a way to consistently meet or volunteer with them.

Don't be afraid to take a look at organizations that reach beyond your hometown or region. There may be a country of ancestry to consider. You may have friends or business contacts in other cities or countries. It's important to maintain these contacts and be connected to people beyond your close friends and family. Some people create a family ancestry tree to learn more about their roots. Others join alumni groups to reach out. There are many ways to stay connected to your community both locally and far away from home. Community connections help you find meaning in a sometimes challenging world and promote longevity, health, and happiness.

◆ ◆ ◆

Valerie is a 46 year old who was concerned about a lump in her breast. I scheduled Valerie for a mammogram and an ultrasound and a biopsy was performed. Unfortunately, this was positive for breast cancer. Valerie subsequently had surgery and chemotherapy to treat her cancer. This was an extremely difficult year for Valerie and her family.

Her surgery was more involved than originally anticipated, and it took nearly a month for her to get her strength back. However, it was the chemotherapy that she found most challenging. Valerie went for chemotherapy infusions every three weeks and the side effects were quite severe. She had limited energy as well nausea and vomiting after most of the treatments. Side effects from the chemotherapy also included severe pain in her knees and hips and neuropathy symptoms including burning pains in her feet. Valerie's oncologist tried different medications to help with these symptoms, but she couldn't take most of them because they caused side effects nearly as bad as the original problems.

With all of these issues, Valerie was unable to do even the most basic of her work and family responsibilities. She took a leave of absence from work. She gave up cooking meals and helping her kids with homework. We often don't think about this, but there are domino effects on each person in the family when one person develops cancer. Valerie's husband did his best to help out, but he had a busy job that required a lot of traveling and they didn't have extended family to help fill in these gaps.

During this time, Valerie's church community provided incredible support. The church created a system to provide dinners for the family and they provided dinners every night for the first six months. The church also created a support system to help drive the kids to their events when Valerie and her husband couldn't do it. When Valerie was weak from chemo and could barely walk, her church community was there to help.

Valerie came back to the office to see me and she spoke glowingly about her church community. She said that she wasn't sure how she could have gotten through everything without them. It was truly inspirational to see a community come together to help a family in need. There are many families living without much extended family support so having a support system like this can be lifesaving. In Valerie's case, it helped get her and her family through a rocky and tumultuous time.

I tell my patients to always keep their eyes open for families in need. This can be within a religious community, at work, at school, or down the street. We live in an interdependent world that starts in our homes and in our local communities. There are people in need on every street, in every neighborhood, in every town and so on.

Find communities that offer support and kindness to others. Join these communities and participate as much as possible. Be sure that you take part in community groups that add a depth of social connection to your life and to the lives of others in your local community and communities around the world.

Habit 39: Find Mentors

When I was a kid, I wanted to be Jimmy Connors. I wanted to have that big booming two-handed backhand. I studied Jimmy's game and modeled my game after his approach to tennis. As I got older and more competitive, several of my tennis coaches also became my role models for becoming a better tennis player. I didn't have nearly the level of talent of Jimmy Connors and I didn't play competitive tennis past high school. However, I learned a powerful lesson during those days—the power of having a mentor.

How does this apply to wellness? You can read everything you can about healthy living, attend lectures, and read every online blog; however, your most effective learning is through real life experience.

You learn best by watching others and practicing what you've observed over and over again. That's why having mentors is so crucial. Do you have mentors in all aspects of your life? Do you have a professional mentor? Do you have a parenting mentor? Do you have mentors for your favorite hobbies? Over the years, I've worked with some incredible doctors who mentored me and helped me to grow in my professional life. I've also had mentors in my family life and in other aspects of life.

Mentors are role models so you can observe how they act, how they prepare, and how they perform. Mentors can be people who you observe from a distance and mentors can be people you know well. If you're fortunate to spend time with your mentors, you can ask them questions to seek their guidance and wisdom. Role modeling is a crucial part of the learning process in all aspects of life. You learn best by watching others and then practicing what you've seen until you have mastered the skill.

This is important because, for good or for bad, you are influenced by those around you. You are affected by the TV shows you watch, the apps you use, the social networks you join, your friends, your family, and the organizations you join. All of these influences affect you: how you feel, how you think and how you develop as a person. No matter how much you resist these influences, human nature dictates that you are influenced by your environment and your community.

I'm a big hockey fan and my favorite team is the Detroit Red Wings. I'm a fan both because I was born in Michigan and also because I admire the way that the team deliberately promotes wellness through the organization. One example of this is the team's approach to mentorship. When a young player joins the Red Wings, the coaching staff assigns the young player to a veteran who knows the Red Wings' approach to training and playing hockey. In other words, they assign each rookie a mentor.

This empowers the veteran whose job it is to teach the younger player all about what it means to be a Red Wing hockey player, while ensuring the new players have an appropriate role model on the team. Their assigned lockers are next to each other so the two players can discuss game preparation, strategy, and whatever else comes up as the season goes on. The young player may struggle with the pressure of the game, the rigorous training schedule, or the sharp glare of being in the public eye. Some young players may not want to discuss an issue with the coaches, so having a fellow player as a mentor ensures that the rookie has someone in whom to confide. This is especially important for personal as well as professional issues that may arise. The Red Wings' mentorship program creates an environment of support and growth that has contributed to the success of the team over the years.

Make mentors a part of your life. You can proactively choose who will influence you or you can let it happen to by chance. I recommend the former. Try your best to find people who will serve as mentors in each aspect of your life. Look to these mentors for wisdom, experience, and guidance. In some circumstances, it can be a person with whom you can meet and talk to for counsel. It could be a more experienced coworker or grandparent who has good judgment and lots of experience. A mentor can guide you at work, with your children, or with your health practices. However, pick your mentors carefully. Think about who might be a good mentor for you in each aspect of your life. Find mentors for your work, family life, friendships, nutrition, exercise, and spiritual practice. Be sure to find people who not only have experience, but also have sound judgment and principles that you respect and want to emulate. Remember that mentors are essentially advisors for your life. Think about this and choose carefully and then speak with each potential mentor and see if he or she might be interested in being a mentor for you.

Listen carefully to your mentors, but also understand that ultimately you need to make your own decisions based on the information that you have and your own judgment. Mentors are trusted advisors, but they shouldn't be making decisions for you. They are there to support and guide you. One of the most important functions of a mentor is to serve as a reminder that you can get through personal or professional challenges as they arise throughout your lifetime.

I recently heard an interview with the great country music singer Vince Gill and he spent much of the interview discussing his mentors. He spoke about those who have influenced him and those whom he continues to look to for sage advice and guidance. He's had huge success in country music and has become a legend in Nashville, yet he still has mentors that help him grow and develop.

Being open to guidance from the right mentors is important as you progress through life. It will serve you well even if you never meet Jimmy Connors.

◆ ◆ ◆

Stephanie is a patient of mine who was severely injured when another driver rear-ended her car. Stephanie was thrown against the steering wheel and suffered serious injuries to her neck and shoulders. I reviewed the medical records from her hospitalization and spoke at length with the orthopedist who was monitoring her recovery. We arranged for Stephanie to have physical therapy and an appropriate exercise program to help with her recovery.

Stephanie and I discussed how she was feeling and she said that she's terrified that she won't regain full strength or range of motion in her shoulders. She asked for advice about what more she could do to support her recovery and the topic of finding a mentor came up. I told her that one of the most important things she could do is to find someone who's been through a similar situation who can mentor her through the recovery process.

Stephanie returned to see me a month later and told me that her physical therapist, Christina, became a physical therapist because she had been through a similar long recovery after a car accident. In addition to helping Stephanie with physical therapy, Christina was helping her cope with the emotions related to her recovery. In a sense,

Christina was Stephanie's mentor. Listening to Stephanie talk, it was clear to me that Christina's guidance was a big help.

———————————— ◆ ◆ ◆ ————————————

Evaluate the areas of your life that would benefit from the guidance of a mentor. Seek out mentors who can help guide you in all aspects of life.

Habit 40: Live Your Values

This habit of *The Wellness Code* is about living your values on a daily basis. In practical terms, this means that your actions reflect your values rather than your emotions. How you interact with others has a direct impact on your health. We all know that negative interactions with others can have a big impact on us. For example, studies have shown that negative interactions with others can increase the risk of heart disease, cancer, autoimmune disease, and many other medical problems. In 2009, researchers from Yale published a study that showed that anger increased the risk of life-threatening abnormal heart rhythms.

We all get angry sometimes, but some of us are able to "bite the bullet" and let it go while others express anger under the banner of "honesty." Numerous studies show that letting difficult emotions dictate your feelings and actions is harmful to your health and longevity. Many people have difficulty stopping themselves from expressing negative thoughts and feelings. When you have a difficult interaction, it's a normal part of the human experience to feel frustration, anger, disappointment, and all sorts of other negative feelings. The challenge is to handle your negative feelings in ways that do not harm you, others, or your relationships. The key to successfully handling difficult feelings and protecting your health is to find practical ways to process these feelings instead of expressing them through your actions. If you need to express your feelings, do so in a constructive way that doesn't add stress to your life.

Whenever you have a negative emotion such as anger, sadness, frustration, or jealousy, the goal is to step back and "observe" the emotion. Don't say or do anything. Don't make a facial expression. Don't write an email. Don't call anyone. It may be very difficult to bite your tongue, but don't do anything yet. Realize that every feeling you experience doesn't always need to be immediately expressed.

When you face one of these feelings, think through how best to respond. Sometimes the best response will be to do nothing. Sometimes, you'll change the topic. Sometimes, you will address the topic currently on the table. Sometimes, you'll want to wait overnight to think about how best to respond.

Your goal is to respond in a way that is consistent with your values. Some people find it works to simply restate what just happened or to guess what the other person may be feeling. For example, if a person behind you at an ATM is getting angry with how long your transaction is taking, he might say to you in a sarcastic tone, "Hey buddy, you think you might be able to go any slower?" You start to feel uncomfortable, even angry. The key is to stop and sit with your thoughts. Don't speak out of anger. If you do, the situation is likely to escalate. You have much better options. You could say nothing, finish up the transaction and move on. If you decide to say something, you could say in a sincere tone, "You must be going somewhere important. I'm so sorry that I'm holding you up." Alternatively, you could say something as simple as, "I'm so sorry this is taking so long."

The key is to resist acting out of negative emotions, but rather to connect with the other person on the level of your values. These are values such as kindness, compassion, and understanding, rather than emotions such as anger, envy, and frustration. Lastly, be careful of tone. Make sure that what you say doesn't have some negative emotions tied up in it. Remember that your actions in the world both towards yourself and towards others should reflect your positive core values.

The next time someone says something rude to you, take a deep breath and don't respond right away. If you choose to respond, do so in a way that seeks connection rather than creates distance through anger or frustration. Respond in a way that is consistent with your values rather than your emotions. The diminished level of confrontation in your life will be good for your heart and your overall health.

Habit 41: Practice Your Faith or Spiritual Practice

In previous habits, I've discussed the importance of staying connected to yourself, your spouse or intimate partner, your children, your friends and family, and your community. Relationships have a big impact on your wellness. There's another connection that is also a major factor in maintaining health and longevity, and that's your spiritual connection. Numerous studies have confirmed that having a spiritual practice has tremendous health benefits.

When you hear the words "spiritual connection," traditional organized religion may immediately spring to mind. However, the health benefits from a spiritual practice can also be achieved outside of traditional organized religions. Other spiritual systems such as twelve-step groups can offer a similar level of health benefit. Many studies validate that having a consistent spiritual practice promotes healthy living.

The remarkable lesson here is that this connection can be found in so many different places. It can be found within an organized religion. It can even be found within a personal relationship with nature or with a hobby such as a musical instrument. Spiritual connection is a complex and mysterious process where something within you connects with a source or "higher power" outside of yourself. This connection builds strength and inspiration for healing and for living a meaningful life.

Each person can practice this spiritual connection is different ways, but it is clear that regularly experiencing this deep connection has tremendous health benefits in terms of healing and optimal health. Scientists will likely be trying for a long time to determine exactly why having a spiritual practice promotes health and longevity. Regardless of why this is the case, the evidence is clear that this is true.

Part of the benefit of practicing spirituality likely derives from the opportunity to connect with others and be supported by others. Part of the benefit is likely because most spiritual practices encourage people to stay away from the bad habits that we know are detrimental to good health such as smoking and excessive alcohol use. However, I would suggest that the power of a spiritual practice goes beyond these practical considerations.

I believe that the profound benefit of spirituality is related to feeling an intangible but trusting, comforting, and guiding connection to a power beyond you that triggers a healing process within the body. This spiritual connection can serve as a bridge to bring you to a healthy, healing place by refocusing your mind, your body, and your soul on the healing mechanisms that already exist within yourself. This process can be considered a sort of antithesis to the reaction you experience to stress. Excessive stress can lead you to lose focus on your priorities and what you know contributes to good health. When you suffer from this stress reaction, many people eat the wrong foods, exercise less, and lose sleep. On the other hand, a healing spiritual practice promotes the thoughts, feelings, and habits that lead to restorative healing.

Think about your spiritual practice, whether it's through a traditional religion, community group, personal hobby, or some other source of spirituality. Find ways to fortify and enrich your spiritual practice.

If you already have a faith with which you're comfortable, find a place of worship and attend services regularly. If you don't have such a faith, try to find another organization or program that provides regular meetings and offers positive support and spiritual guidance. Look for spiritual communities that involve both individual and community practices. Become a consistent participant in a spiritual program that is based on principles consistent with your values.

Habit 42: Let Go of Emotional Pain from the Past

Unresolved emotional pain from the past is one of the most significant contributing factors to current physical and psychological health problems. The internal pain of disappointment and loss creates an emotional and spiritual process within your mind and body that greatly impacts your wellness. It impacts both your physical and emotional state. Thus, constructively processing past pain is so very important for your health.

For the purposes of this habit, it's helpful to find a word for this past emotional pain and that word is grief. I define grief as the current physical and emotional manifestations of one or more experiences from the past. Most families and most schools don't teach children the tools and strategies needed to handle grief. They don't provide tools and strategies to process painful experiences. Thus, most children and adults end up avoiding or repressing painful experiences. Of course, this is only a short-term solution which serves to bury the pain rather than deal with it. This inevitably leads to problems down the road when this unresolved grief boils up and spills over creating current day health problems. This internal stress may manifest itself in marital or work problems. It may trigger intestinal problems. It may contribute to high blood pressure or diabetes. It can contribute to an endless number of medical problems.

Avoiding grief through denial or repression or other strategies may make you feel better in the short-term, but these are not effective long-term strategies. Each of these options will cause problems unless you set aside time to process your pain and loss. If grief is not processed correctly, it will linger in the body and in the mind and the stress that this creates can be profound. It suppresses the immune system, making you more vulnerable to infections and other health problems. It predisposes you to inflammation which is at the root of problems such as autoimmune diseases, vascular disease, and cancers.

Let's focus on how children handle grief. As a child, feelings of grief can be truly terrifying. It can feel just like the world is closing in and there's no escape. So what can a child do? These emotions are often so difficult that children feel the need to do whatever possible to get rid of these feelings. Some of the psychological tools that children use to process pain are strategies like repression, denial, projection and displacement. Unfortunately, these tools are usually ineffective and lead to symptoms such as anger, depression, anxiety, or isolation.

For example, if a child is mourning the loss of a friendship, he or she might become angry at a sibling or parent. Alternatively, he might begin to believe that a friend is angry at him rather than dealing with his own pain and sadness related to missing his friend. The child might retreat into denial and lose touch with the fact that he has any unpleasant feelings. Repression might occur where the feelings are buried deep in the child's mind. All of these are common strategies that children use to hide from, mask, and escape from pain and disappointment. In the short term, these strategies can make a child feel better, but the problem is that all of this unresolved pain can continue to mount. If this process continues for a long period of time, the child can end up with a tremendous amount of unresolved pain deeply rooted in his or her psyche.

What happens to these children after years of repressing, denying, projection, and displacing all of this pain? Sadly, some people end up using alcohol or drugs to mask and escape from these feelings. Some end up acting out and end up in prison. The final result is rarely a positive outcome.

Unresolved pain, otherwise known as grief, is at the root of many adult problems and can have a profound effect on wellness. Many decades after the initial event, that pain is still deep inside having been buried so many years ago. This unresolved grief can aggravate and trigger many an endless array of health problems including intestinal problems, heart disease, autoimmune disease, and many other problems.

What can be done about this? There are two main steps to consider. These steps are:

1. *Recognize and process past emotional pain*
2. *Recognize and process new emotional pain*

The first step in healing any problem is recognition. Recognize that grief can occur when you experience a loss. Think back on your past, and get in touch with situations that may still be affecting you today. Keeping a journal can be very helpful. The next time that you suffer a significant loss, whether it is a relationship, a job, or the loss of a loved one, recognize that this is a truly significant loss. Remember that a loss needs to be addressed and processed.

In addition to keeping a journal, one of the most important tools to let the past go is meditation (habit 20). With meditation, you focus on the present moment. When your mind drifts into the past or future, gently release your thoughts and return your focus and attention to the present moment.

The third tool is meeting with a therapist, but be sure to find one who spends most of the time helping you live better today rather than overanalyzing the past. A good therapist helps you to understand the past, but doesn't encourage blaming others for current problems. It is important to understand the past, but live in the now. If emotional pain is affecting you physically or emotionally, consider working with a licensed, health professional to process this loss and learn how to integrate the past into your current life. If one-on-one counselling isn't right for you, group sessions such as a 12-step group can also be of tremendous value.

Never resort to alcohol or drugs to deal with grief. If this is something you are struggling with, a wonderful book to read that touches on alcohol and loss is a book called *Drinking: A Love Story* by Caroline Knapp. It's an insightful book about how people use alcohol to deal with emotional pain and the devastating effects that can occur when grief isn't effectively handled. Don't run away from the pain of loss. Grieve those losses so you can move on in your life, changed by the loss that you've experienced but emotionally whole and healthy nonetheless.

$$\diamond \diamond \diamond$$

Ellen is a 46 year old television executive who came to see me because of her psoriasis. She has a long history of skin problems related to her psoriasis which flares up when she's sleep deprived or under a lot of stress. I prescribed medications for the psoriasis and then I asked her about her stress level and sleep habits to see if there was a trigger for her symptoms. She said that she was having a fairly uneventful year with just typical family and work stress. I then asked her if anything out of the ordinary had happened in the last five years.

Ellen paused and told me that her husband died three years ago. The way Ellen spoke implied that she had seemingly moved past her active grief. Ellen appeared without emotion as she told me about her college sweetheart and their marriage. It wasn't until I asked about her three children that I saw the kinks in her armor. She got a lump in her throat and began to cry as she started to tell me more.

She told me that she went back to work three days after her husband's death. She said that she coped with the loss by submerging herself in work and didn't seek any counseling or any support. She said her family was amazed at how well she persevered and how she put her children first. I didn't say much as this was Ellen's chance to open her heart and share her experience, pain and unresolved grief.

Losing a spouse is like having open-heart surgery. And just as she wouldn't think of going back to work three days after open heart surgery, going back to work so quickly really wasn't best for her after losing her husband. Healing from such a profound loss takes time. This grief leaves a heavy toll on the body, mind, and soul and needs to be properly processed. If not, it will continue to manifest itself in all sorts of harmful ways. In this case, the unresolved pain was still affecting her, and was possibly contributing to the problems she was having with psoriasis.

I told Ellen that the medications would help with the psoriasis, but that she should consider finding a therapist or a support group to help her process the grief that she had kept buried for three years. In effect, the psoriasis was just the tip of the iceberg of her unresolved grief. I gave her the phone numbers of some excellent local therapists and the contact numbers for local support groups and asked her return to see me in a couple of weeks to follow-up on how she's doing.

◈ ◈ ◈

Habit 43: Live Within Your Means

Living within your means may be one of the most relevant habits for current times. So many people are currently drowning in debt. It has become commonplace to spend more than you make to try to live the lifestyle you see in magazines or on television.

For generations, purchasing only what you could afford was the way most people in the Western world lived. However, in the 20th century, the "credit card mentality" began. This effectively expanded the amount of money that people believed to be at their disposal. It used to be that people only went into debt to purchase a home. Now, using credit to buy everyday items such as restaurant meals, clothes, and vacations has become commonplace.

Of course, modern history shows how this overzealous credit expansion led to the economic downturn in 2008. I saw firsthand how this can affect both the global economy and individual families. It wasn't pretty.

After the market crash of 2008, I saw patient after patient struggling with the health consequences of the stress of their financial situation. Financial instability, particularly living above and beyond one's means, creates tremendous levels of stress. Studies confirm that high levels of stress related to financial debt contribute to drug and alcohol addiction, sleep disorders, headaches, blood pressure issues, heart attack risk, and many other serious health-related problems.

It's important to be careful with financial expenditures to safeguard your financial future and your health. This means that you should plan purchases based on what your budget allows. You should try to not exceed your budget and to avoid purchasing too many items with credit. Every individual or family should have a budget and stick to it.

Create an individual or family budget and make sure that you keep it balanced each month. Be realistic and prepare for emergencies. It's ideal to have an emergency fund equal to six to twelve months of living expenses just in case you unexpectedly lose a job or have unanticipated medical expenses.

Some people purchase a large house or an expensive car because they anticipate that future raises and promotions will make paying for those items easy. Although it may appear that you'll have the resources to pay something back down the road, it's generally best not to overcommit just in case your financial situation should change for the worse. Even if it does turn out that you can meet your debt payments, most people still experience unnecessary stress—and subsequent health consequences—from the experience of being in debt.

Make the decision to live within your means. That means that, except for rare exceptions, only make purchases that you can afford without borrowing money. When the time comes to get a new car, review your finances and see what you can afford. If your finances allow it, you may be able to purchase that new car. However, the numbers may indicate that you need to buy a used car to stay within your budget. You may decide that it's best to purchase a less expensive used car even though you could afford the new car. Living within your means will do more than balance your budget and keep you out of excessive debt. It will significantly help you to avoid the stress that can disrupt and destroy your health.

Do your best to keep your expenditures within your budget and to avoid buying things on credit. The immediate result of living this way is that you may not be able to purchase everything that you want. It may mean that your vacations aren't quite as nice as you would prefer. It may mean that you move into a slightly smaller house. Living within your means can be difficult because it involves sacrificing short-term pleasure for long-term gain. By making prudent financial decisions now, you're safeguarding yourself from the stress that debt that can create. You're prioritizing your wellness.

Habit 44: Practice Integrity

What you say to people and what you promise people should be as strong as oak. Research has shown that being authentic to your word promotes good health. One study from England published in *The Journal of Counseling Psychology* found less depression and more contentment in life for those who are more authentic and true to their word. The power of integrity comes from having a core set of principles that you follow and honor. Integrity is about having your actions and your words be truthful, authentic, and real.

In today's world, many do not always practice this habit. Some people stretch the truth and overstate accomplishments. Doing this is simply not good for you as it promotes a false sense of identity. It creates a discordant feeling when your public identity clashes with your true authentic identity. This disparity between your false self and your authentic true self leads to internal stress. This ultimately manifests itself as a destructive energy within your body that is detrimental to your health.

You hear Hollywood celebrities talk about the stress of trying to be someone they're not and the difficulty of trying to live up to the public persona created by gossip magazines and publicists. This kind of inconsistency between who you are and how others see you creates an internal stress, which can lead to alcoholism, drug addiction, and a physical toll on your mind and body. This toll can ultimately contribute to damage to your arteries, which can lead to heart attacks and strokes. It can even damage the DNA of your cells, which can predispose you to develop cancer. It can contribute to damage to your immune system and can contribute to autoimmune diseases such as rheumatoid arthritis, type 1 diabetes, and psoriasis.

Integrity allows your actions and words to flow naturally from your true authentic self. It creates an environment where there is no discordance between how the world sees you and how you see yourself. Your goal should be to live your life in a way that is consistent with your values so you don't create potentially damaging internal stress.

In addition to the health benefits of practicing integrity, there are also practical benefits. Your relationships are stronger when your friends and family members know they can count on you. When someone is a no-show for an event or doesn't do something they promised to do, the result is a loss of trust. Relationships with children are impacted by whether or not a promise is kept, just like in the classic Harry Chapin song "Cat's In The Cradle."

The goal is to live your life so that your words, actions, and commitments are in line with your authentic self. When you give someone a promise, they know they can rely on your word. When you commit to something, others can count on you. Practicing integrity on a consistent basis is a crucial habit for healthy living and one that you should strive to uphold every day. Make it a practice to honor what you say and what you promise. Only make commitments that you can keep and keep the commitments you make.

Habit 45: Leave a Legacy

Leaving a legacy means different things to different people. To me, it means that each person should leave something behind that continues to touch the world long after you're gone. Every single one of us is wired for creativity; we just have to tap into it. You are wired to create things that didn't exist before. Songwriters do this when they write a song. They put different notes, melodies, and lyrics together and a new song is created that can touch people's hearts. Filmmakers do this when they create a movie that continues to affect people decades after its release.

You don't need to make movies or write songs to be creative and leave a legacy. You have the potential to create something special related to your family, your work, or your hobbies. Legacies are important because they create powerful connections between generations. We also know that these connections help relieve stress and promote healing within yourself and within your family. Feeling connected to others provides important nurturing mechanisms to the human body.

What sort of legacy do you want to create? One way to leave a legacy is to build a family and create lives and relationships that will carry on into the future. Raising a child is a creative process that leaves a vitally important legacy. If you are blessed to have children, you spend years teaching, molding, and instructing them. If you're fortunate, years later a wonderful person emerges into adulthood prepared to have a productive life. This is a form of creation that leaves a legacy behind that will continue to impact the world long after you're gone. In this sense, leaving a legacy is the ultimate form of extending your longevity.

Think about ways that you can practice your creativity. Perhaps you have a hobby where you can be creative. Hopefully, your home or work life provide opportunities. It's important to find areas where you can be creative and find new ways to experience life. Ask any expert on Alzheimer's disease and they'll tell you that one of the most important strategies to enhance and support memory is to continue to challenge the mind through creativity. Being a creator literally provides exercise for your mind. Challenge yourself to be a creator. Challenge yourself to create a legacy.

Tyler is a 51 year old high school science teacher with type 2 diabetes who recently suffered a heart attack. Fortunately, his heart attack was relatively mild. He recovered quickly and was back to work within a couple of months. Tyler came to see me to follow-up on his heart issues and review his medical condition.

After a thorough medical evaluation, I concluded that Tyler was doing quite well in his recovery from the heart attack. Tyler was doing well at work and was settling back into his responsibilities as a teacher. However, I also learned that he wasn't entirely satisfied with his current professional situation. During his hospitalization, Tyler had a lot of time to think about his priorities, his past achievements, and what he wants to accomplish in the future. Although Tyler loves teaching and is still fascinated with science, he described feeling somewhat bored at work.

Tyler and I had a long discussion about his values and the importance of finding meaning and passion in his work. Tyler said that things have gotten repetitive at work and he finds much less fulfillment now as compared to twenty years ago. Tyler was thinking about going back to school for a new degree or perhaps leaving teaching and trying something else. From our discussions, it was clear that teaching, in and of itself, was still a passion for Tyler. He simply had gotten into a rut at work and needed to find some new inspiration—some new motivation. I explained to him that being a creator is so important and I asked him if there's a way for him to create something new related to his work.

All of a sudden, Tyler had a spark in his eyes and he started to think of ideas that might work for him. He mentioned his love of teaching and he said that he has considered writing a book on teaching. He also mentioned possibly starting a podcast about some of the topics that he covers in his science classes. He also had the idea of starting a tutoring company. Ideas were flowing from him as we sorted through all the possibilities. It was now clear that Tyler didn't need to change his entire career—he just needed to shift his perspective and his attention onto the creative process. He needed to shift from going through the motions to being a proactive creator. Later that year, Tyler called to let me know that he was finishing a book on teaching, and I was thrilled to hear that. The energy and passion in his voice made it clear that he had found a renewed excitement and joy for life.

◆ ◆ ◆

How can you be a creator? Think through your life and find ways to be creative. Do you like to cook? If so, create new and interesting recipes. Do you play an instrument? Try your hand at writing a song. Do you like to write? Try writing a poem or a short story or a screenplay. Do you like technology? Try to design an app or start a podcast. Do you like to travel? Start a travel website or blog to help others find interesting places to visit. Have you had a major life-altering experience about which you have become an expert? Start a website or a blog about that topic. There are so many ways to be creative. Find ways that work for you. Find topics that interest you and keep you motivated. Spend some quality time thinking about this and then create, create, create.

Habit 46: Visualize Before You Act

Decisions, decisions, decisions. We all make decisions each and every day. Some decisions are simple, like what kind of coffee to order or what movie to see this weekend. Some decisions are more complicated and more important such as which career to pursue, how many children to have, which job to take, where to live, or whom you should marry.

Some decisions are life-altering and others are fairly inconsequential. That being said, I see people struggle every day with decision-making. Take a new job or stay with your current job? Move to Boston, Chicago, Dallas, Los Angeles or Atlanta? Do the taxes or clean the house? There are so many options in life; making a choice can be paralyzing to people who don't know how to approach decisions.

Unfortunately, little time and attention is paid to teaching people how to make good, sound decisions that promote a healthy life. Your decisions in life directly relate to your wellness so it's extremely important to know how to make effective decisions. Each choice you make affects your stress level, which directly impacts so many aspects of health and ultimately your longevity.

To help you, I'd like to present a habit that is useful for making sound decisions. It is a way to look at your options and to use your feelings and experiences to guide you to pick the best choice for you.

This is how it works: let's say you have two job offers. Call them Job A and Job B. You spend days and weeks getting information about the two jobs. You've analyzed every aspect of the two jobs. Perhaps you've even made a chart of the pros and cons of each job. You have all the necessary information to fully understand the two jobs, but you still aren't sure which one to choose.

Try sitting down and performing the following experiential exercise. Close your eyes and pretend that you've already taken Job A. You close your eyes and pretend that you've already made the choice. You've taken Job A and turned down Job B. How does it feel? How does it feel to have made that commitment? Do you feel good about the decision? You might be nervous about the new job, but do you feel good about the decision? Focus on how you feel about the decision that you made. Do you feel confident that you made the right choice for you and your family and that the decision was consistent with your values, priorities, and life plans? Alternatively, do you feel regret and disappointment over your choice? Do you wish you had chosen Job B and feel like you've made the wrong choice?

Once you've visualized yourself having made the decision, all of the consequences that would result from that choice will be become clear in your mind. Search your mind and your heart. Try to experience your thoughts and your feelings and see if you feel at peace that you made the correct choice. Typically, when you make the correct choice, you feel peace. You feel good about your decision. You may be nervous about how things will go, but there's peace in knowing that the correct decision was made. An uncomfortable, unsettled feeling creeps into your mind when you've made the wrong choice. Search your mind and your heart to see if you have a feeling of peace or discontent.

Once you finish this process with Job A, perform the same exercise with Job B. Pretend that you've chosen Job B. Go through the same mental exercise of visualizing your life after you have chosen Job B and follow the same process that I just discussed. Sometimes you have to perform this exercise several times, but usually you will know which the right decision is.

If you try this process and don't have a clear feeling about which is the correct choice, then there are four possibilities.

First, you may not have enough information about your choices. If that's the case, then go back and learn more about the two options. Ask more questions. Think more deeply about the short term and long term prospects with each choice and the effects this may have on you and your loved ones.

The second possibility is that the two choices are literally a toss-up. They're so comparable that they may be equivalent.

The third possibility is that neither choice is correct for you. This would indicate that you need to look for another option.

The fourth possibility is that you didn't fully engage in this exercise, which means that you didn't fully experience the thoughts and feelings related to having accepted each job. If that's the case, go back and try the exercise again.

This process can be incredibly helpful with decision making for both minor and major situations in life. For major decisions, it's sometimes a good idea to engage your closest friends and family in this process. They often can help predict how it will feel for you to make each decision as they know your priorities and your goals.

The key here is to fully engage in this experiential exercise. When faced with a new decision, visualize yourself having made each choice. Write down your thoughts and feelings if you find that helpful. Fully imagine and think through how it would feel to have made each decision and get in touch with the thoughts and emotions related to each decision. By doing so, the right decision should crystallize and the optimal path should become clear. Once you get in the habit of doing this visualization exercise, you will find yourself automatically taking this step any time you are faced with a decision.

Habit 47: Practice Gratitude: The Secret to Happiness

We are all grateful to a certain extent. We may appreciate having a home, a job, friends and family. However, sometimes we focus on what we wish we had rather than all the blessings that we do have.

This tendency has been made more extreme by the proliferation of magazines and websites dedicated to showing you how others live. Instead of comparing your life to your neighbors, you now have the ability to literally see how your lifestyle compares to that of the rich and famous all over the world. This often leads to dissatisfaction with what you have and unrealistic expectations of how your life should be lived.

What if you took the practice of gratitude and made it a habit to practice it each day? Tall order, huh? What would happen if you became truly grateful for every moment of your life? What if you appreciated opening your eyes in the morning, seeing the sun rise, having that morning cup of coffee or tea, going for a walk, hearing the sound of birds chirping, and seeing your loved ones? No matter how difficult your life may be, everyone has so much for which to be thankful. The secret, though, is to find ways to have this perspective as often as possible.

Gratitude happens when you focus on all the wonderful things that happen each day rather than think about everything that "goes wrong." With gratitude, you choose to appreciate every moment of your life. If you focus on the beauty in life, you will experience a completely different state of mind.

You could even appreciate aspects of the moments that don't seem so wonderful on the surface. For example, can you be grateful for having a disagreement with a neighbor? Is that even possible? Well, it takes practice and effort, but you can try to see disagreements as serving some higher purpose. Perhaps it will encourage you to foster better community relations in your neighborhood or to grow as a person and practice understanding another's perspective. Perhaps it allows you to model for your kids how to accept other people's differing perspectives.

Another example of a less obvious opportunity to practice gratitude is when you're standing in line in the grocery store and the person in front of you is struggling to write a check and is taking a long time. You have a decision to make. Do you get impatient and express your frustration to the people around you? Another choice would be to focus on the fact that you're about to purchase delicious food and that your financial circumstances allow you to do so without stress.

In any moment, you can choose to focus on either the blessings or the curses in life. This is a challenge as it's easy to focus on what's wrong in life—the glass being half-empty rather than half-full. If your car looks perfect in every way except for one tiny scratch on the driver's side door, do you focus on that scratch or on the fact that you have a reliable car that enables you to more easily live your life?

Try to focus your attention on what's great in life and be grateful for the blessings that come your way every day. The key here is to experience gratitude in all aspects of life whenever possible. It shifts your perspective from one of frustration and unhappiness to harmony, acceptance, and happiness.

One great life lesson is that gratitude is the key to happiness.

When you focus mainly on problems, you experience stress which wears on your body, mind, and spirit. On the other hand, when you focus on all the blessings in life, you experience happiness and fulfillment.

Gratitude is often discussed as a virtue, something good for your soul. It turns out that gratitude is also good for your physical and emotional health. One of my favorite studies was the University of California Davis Medical Center study where patients were instructed to write down the five best things that happened to them each day, while another group was instructed to write down the five worst things, and a third group had to write down any five things that happened that day. After twelve weeks, the researchers concluded that the first group (the gratitude group) was happier, had fewer health complaints, and even slept better than the other two groups. Fascinating, right? Focusing on the positive things that happen to you is good for your health.

That's not to say that you should simply be a Pollyanna and ignore problems that need to be addressed. You need to deal with problems, but they shouldn't be your main focus. If you have a tendency to focus on the negative in life, you may need to force yourself to focus on the positive. Gratitude works because it encourages happiness in life and is the secret sauce to wellness.

What is happiness? Happiness is the state of mind that results from experiencing life with appreciation and gratitude. Happiness is simply a state of mind just as envy, jealously, frustration, or anger are states of mind. Happiness is a state of mind that anyone can attain if the proper practices of gratitude are followed.

On the other hand, unhappiness is the result of struggling with life and finding anger and frustration with each moment. Unhappiness arises when you see challenges as struggles rather than what they truly are: opportunities for growth. Rather than seeing life as a struggle, try to see life as the grand experience that it is and appreciate all the blessings that come your way.

When you think about this, it makes sense. You're happy when you appreciate what's happening in your life. When you resist your life, you will tend to be unhappy. Take a moment and remember to practice gratitude every day. Make gratitude a part of your life and the lives that you touch. Every moment is an opportunity to be grateful for what is going right. It is up to each person to decide whether or not to seize the opportunity to be grateful and experience happiness.

There are many wonderful resources that can help you practice happiness on a daily basis. *Happify.com* is a website and app with loads of helpful strategies. *LiveHappy.com* is another useful website that that publishes a magazine and a podcast.

◈ ◈ ◈

Emily is a 52 year old patient who was once a rising star at a financial services company. Just as she was up for a promotion to vice president, Emily was diagnosed with stage 3 breast cancer. This is an advanced stage of breast cancer. After receiving her diagnosis, Emily reluctantly decided to give up her work and focus on regaining her health. Emily endured multiple surgeries and numerous rounds of chemotherapy and had done well from a cancer standpoint. When she came to see me as a patient, the cancer was in remission, as her recent testing showed no evidence of active cancer.

However, Emily reported that she was struggling in other areas of her life. Even though she was happy to be alive, she felt lost inside. She had lost her joy and zest for life that was such an integral part of her personality. She told me that she felt worthless and unhappy most of the time. Emily and I discussed her feelings in depth and, after much discussion, decided to start her on an anti-depressant. However, we also discussed other strategies to focus her attention in ways that promote happiness. In particular, we discussed gratitude.

At first, Emily said she had little for which to be grateful. She spoke about losing her career. She spoke about her strained relationship with her sister. She spoke about her marriage, which had lost its passion. I asked Emily if there's anything in her life that's a blessing and for which she is grateful. Emily paused and then said that she was grateful to be alive.

I asked her to keep a gratitude journal and that each day she should list five things for which she's grateful. Emily agreed and she called me a month later to share some insights that she had. She said focusing on the blessings in life had inspired her to reach out to her friends and that she was going for a thirty minute walk each morning with her friend Maggie. She also said that she had reached out to her sister and they had lunch together. She said that she was starting to get back into tennis and that she was feeling stronger. She sounded much more vibrant, which was a noticeable shift for her in a positive direction.

◈ ◈ ◈

There are specific tools and strategies that can help to create an attitude of gratitude. The following nine tools are particularly effective in promoting gratitude and happiness within yourself and those that you encounter. Read through these practices and see which ones work for you.

1. Gratitude Journal

A gratitude journal is a journal where you write down what you appreciate about your life. You can journal in your smart phone, tablet or computer. Alternatively, you can use an old-fashioned paper journal. One of the best ways to use a gratitude journal is to make an entry each morning upon arising. Each morning, list three things for which you're grateful, whether it's a person, place, or thing. It could be something recent, in the past or something happening right now. Try to make sure that at least one of your items is new to your gratitude journal. It is important to list at least one new item a day as it forces you to continue to find new things to appreciate.

You could even try to find ways to appreciate things that didn't go your way. For example, let's say your favorite football team lost a big game on Sunday. What could you find to appreciate about the loss? Perhaps the loss might inspire your team to focus and play harder in the playoffs or perhaps it may help secure a better draft pick in the next college player draft. Use your gratitude journal on a daily basis.

2. **Gratitude Prayer**

Most major religions or spiritual practices teach the power of prayer. Many people use prayer to ask for something, whether for forgiveness or for the speedy recovery of a friend having surgery. However, some prayers are about gratitude. Think about the prayers that are typically recited at religious ceremonies, before dinner or during special events. Most of those prayers are about gratitude. Yes, good old gratitude; being thankful for something.

It can be a prayer of thankfulness for having enough food, good health or for all sorts of other things. I would venture to say that most traditional prayers are, at their core, prayers of gratitude or thankfulness. That's one of the core benefits of a healthy spiritual practice. It's an organized way to practice gratitude. Prayer can be private within your heart and mind. Prayer could also be public in the setting of organized religion or some other community group. The key here is that prayer can be a profound, sometimes spiritual way to express thankfulness, appreciation, and gratitude whether it's private or public. Thus, the second tool for gratitude is to recite a prayer of thankfulness.

3. **Gratitude Walk**

When walking and gratitude are combined together, you get the gratitude walk. How does this work? Go for a walk and use a step counter to count your steps just as I discussed in habit 16. However, on a gratitude walk, find something to appreciate every thousand steps that you take, which is about every half a mile. You can use a fitness tracker from FitBit, Jawbone, Apple, Garmin, Withings, or Basis to track your steps, or you can use one of the many smartphone step tracking apps.

As you walk, look for things to appreciate. For example, I tend to go for walks along the hills and mountains near my house so I see so many beautiful parts of nature from plants to trees to birds to the ocean in the distance. There is so much beauty to appreciate in such a bucolic setting, but you can find something to appreciate no matter where you are.

As you walk, make it a habit to find something to appreciate every 1,000 steps (or about every half mile). This is a great daily exercise and daily meditative process. Think about how a walk rooted in appreciation helps to center your mind and heart in feelings of gratitude that promote good health.

After you've done a few gratitude walks, I recommend planning your walks to visit places to actually give thanks to people. Perhaps you can take a walk to your grocery store, dry cleaner, coffee shop, or pharmacy and thank the people that work there. You will be amazed at how much this means to people.

Can you imagine how good it feels to have someone walk into your store simply to thank you? In addition, you will be amazed at how good this feels for you. Expressing your appreciation will improve the quality of your day and fill your heart with feelings of joy and happiness. If you don't live close enough to walk to these stores, then consider a "gratitude drive" where you can drive to these places. Of course, a drive won't give you the same health benefits as a walk, but the act of expressing your gratitude will still be beneficial.

4. Gratitude Meditation

As we've discussed before, meditation is a practice where you focus your attention on a word, phrase, or movement and give your conscious mind a short vacation. You focus on one thing— it could be your breath, a prayer, a mantra, or even just your hands. The key to meditation is to spend a period of time focused on something and, when your mind begins to wonder to thoughts about the past or future, you let those thoughts go and bring your attention back to the present moment.

There are many studies now showing that meditation can help in so many different ways from improved sleep to reduced stress to improved blood pressure control. Given all the impressive health benefits of meditation, what would happen if you combined the power of meditation with gratitude? The key to meditation is to maintain your attention for a sustained period of time. Let's say that you decide that each day you would spend five minutes meditating on something for which you are grateful, perhaps for having two children. Find a quiet place to sit down and do your meditation and focus on being grateful for your children. Your attention and your concentration will stay on a mental image of your children and all the many reasons why you're grateful that they're a part of your life. When other thoughts begin to intrude into your meditation, you passively release those thoughts and return to being grateful for your children. Tomorrow you might pick someone or something else to use in your gratitude meditation. You might pick your car or your home or having enough food to eat for breakfast. The focus of your gratitude mediation can vary from day to day each day. However, be sure to find time for this on a regular basis. The gratitude meditation is a powerful and meaningful way to combine two useful tools into one extraordinarily powerful daily practice.

5. Gratitude Letter To Yourself

This is similar to a gratitude journal, but instead of keeping a journal, the idea is to sit down and write a good old-fashioned letter to your past self. Each week, write a letter to yourself at some time in the past—at seven years old or thirty years old or whatever age you like—and express some gratitude in the letter. Looks back at those days from the past and find things for which to be thankful. What could you write? Try to reflect back on how the choices you made at that age have helped you in life or taught you a lesson that has been useful to you. You can also give yourself some wisdom or some sage advice that you have learned over the years. The focus of these letters should be on appreciating things that happened to you and things that you did for others.

It's also important to give some comfort and compassion to yourself for the times when you might have needed it. Let's say that you struck out in a big baseball game when you were 10 years old. Let's say that you didn't have a date to the senior prom back in high school. We all can recall moments in our lives when we struggled with something or had a bad experience. Write a letter to help yourself get through that tough time and try to find some appreciation for what happened. What would you write in your gratitude letters? What wisdom would you impart to yourself during the past? The gratitude letter can be extremely powerful as it expands your awareness of your own struggles. It allows you the opportunity to see yourself from a new perspective and enrich your heart with self-compassion and self-love.

6. **Gratitude Dinner**

Dining together as a family can be a wonderful way to express gratitude. This is an activity I encourage families to practice every night if possible. Some families recite a religious or spiritual prayer as part of the practice. Alternatively, some families simply go around the table and have each person say one thing they appreciate about the meal. The key is to encourage each family member to focus on appreciating life and the blessings of the meal.

7. **Gratitude Social Media Post**

How can you use social media platforms to encourage appreciation? You can write a gratitude social media post. This can be done by simply posting a thank you message. Those who want to be creative can use audio or video to craft their post. The key is to express public gratitude for something, someone, or some organization.

Recently I used Twitter to show my appreciation for a singer whose music I've enjoyed for decades. I sent out a tweet of gratitude to the singer expressing how much I appreciate the great work that she has created. Soon after I shared that tweet, I received a reply from the singer thanking me for my words of gratitude. It was clear from her reply that my tweet had meant a lot to her. At the time, I realized that this exchange of tweets also meant a lot to me, because it encouraged a feeling of appreciation in my heart. The exchange helped to make my day and I suspect it may have made her day a little brighter as well.

Think of ways that you can use social media to give thanks. Pick your favorite social media platform and make it a regular practice to send a message of thanks to people you appreciate.

Keep it sweet and keep it simple. Be honest and be specific about why you're thankful and how this person has enriched your life. Social media isn't always used for enriching purposes, but make this a consistent practice for you. You will be surprised and amazed at how much these sorts of messages mean to others. You will also be amazed how much it means to you.

8. Gratitude Letter

This may be my favorite gratitude exercise. For this exercise, think of someone to whom you want to give thanks. It can be someone from your current life or someone from your past. A gratitude letter can be especially meaningful when you reach out to someone who may not be aware of the impact they had on you. It could be a teacher from elementary school or a friend from years ago or perhaps someone who helped you with something. It can be someone who you see all the time, like a waiter at your favorite restaurant or your dentist. Write that person a note—either an email or, better yet, a good old-fashioned letter. Keep it brief, but let them know that you appreciate them and explain why you're thankful for whatever role they played in your life. Occasionally I will receive a gratitude letter from a patient or family member of a patient. It always means a lot to me. Make writing a gratitude note a regular practice.

9. Random Acts of Kindness

One of the best ways to promote gratitude and happiness within yourself and within your family is to regularly perform random acts of kindness. Many religions teach about compassion and kindness to others and there's a reason for that. In addition to helping others, kindness promotes a feeling of gratitude and appreciation within yourself. Make it a practice to show kindness to others as often as possible. You can show kindness in a smile or a pleasant comment. You can show kindness in doing a favor for someone in need. You can also show kindness to a stranger, which is a particularly powerful source of gratitude. As discussed in habit 36, you can purchase a cup of coffee or tea for the person behind you in line at your local coffee shop. Random acts of kindness promote your own happiness and also help to spread wellness to others.

These nine gratitude practices can help increase your feelings of appreciation. If you are able to incorporate some of these ideas into your life on a consistent basis, you will be surprised at how much more happiness you feel and spread to others. Give one or more of these gratitude tools a try and see what works for you. Find ways to integrate gratitude practices into your daily life. Find a time and a place where you will practice some form of gratitude every day. Finding ways to incorporate these tools into your everyday life can be a life changing practice. Every moment is an opportunity to appreciate all the wonderful parts of life. It is up to you to decide whether or not to seize that opportunity.

Habit 48: The Power of Music

Most people enjoy listening to music and can easily name their favorite bands and songs. However, music can be more than just a fun activity. Music can also provide tremendous health, emotional, and even spiritual benefits.

————————◆ ◆ ◆————————

Health Benefits of Music

1. Reduces pain
2. Promotes focus
3. Improves mood
4. Improves motivation
5. Improves cognitive skills such as visual and verbal skills
6. Improved exercise performance
7. Reduces anxiety
8. Supports the immune system
9. Improves memory
10. Improves blood circulation
11. Improves recovery from cancer treatments
12. Improves discipline in food choices
13. Improves recovery from exercise
14. Improves recovery from surgery
15. Improves blood pressure
16. Improves recovery from strokes
17. Improves sleep

————————◆ ◆ ◆————————

Many people find that listening to music while exercising makes the experience more enjoyable. For example, I watch music performances on my tablet while I use the elliptical trainer. The music helps keep me motivated and consistent with my exercise routine. Moreover, calm and peaceful music can be incredibly helpful to maintain attention and focus while meditating (habit 20).

In addition to making it easier to exercise and meditate, there is compelling evidence that listening to music can provide measurable health benefits. Studies have shown that music therapy can help patients recover from heart attacks. Music has been shown to help children develop visual skills, communication skills, and language skills. Music has also been shown to help improve memory in patients suffering from dementia and to help patients recover from surgery. Music helps people suffering from insomnia, stress-related disorders, and chronic pain. In addition to these benefits, some fascinating studies have even shown that music can help improve the function of the immune system. It's clear that music has the ability to tap into your body's natural healing mechanisms and help in many different ways.

Apart from helping with physical health problems, music can also provide emotional benefits—music can make the fun times even more fun and the painful times a little less painful. Historically, music has been a prominent part of most every culture, and there's a reason for that. One of my hobbies is to host a music review podcast called Five Minute Music Reviews where we review albums. We also feature some amazing cancer charities that help patients and their families through the ordeal of cancer. In my practice, I've heard many patients tell me that music helped them get through some pretty dark times: the loss of a loved one, a job loss, divorce, or other challenges they have faced. Music helps. There are songs that still remind you of a time and a feeling from many years ago. When a song like this comes on the radio, it takes you back to that exact moment when something happened to you; it almost feels like you're right there in that moment all over again with the same feelings and the same emotions fresh in your heart and mind.

Music has such a profound effect on people because it taps into your deepest emotions. By helping you connect with those emotions, music gives you the chance to heal what lies buried deep inside. As we discussed in habit 42, pain that has been buried deep inside and not properly processed often leads to using alcohol or drugs to escape from these feelings. This is the root of so many health problems that adults struggle with long after they have left childhood. The emotional pain creeps out just like garbage from an overstuffed garbage can. Even in adulthood, it's still important to make sure your past emotional pain has been processed. If not, it will affect you in ways that negatively impact your current life situation.

Life is about experiencing the full range of your emotions and staying in touch with these emotions rather than burying this treasure deep inside of you. That's one of the secrets of emotional health. Sometimes you go through the motions of going to work or taking care of the kids, but spend little time or attention on your feelings. It's far easier in the short-term to avoid thinking about what's troubling you and to keep those feelings buried away. However, do you know what happens when your feelings get ignored for too long? They will eventually explode later in life—usually in a not so good way.

This is why music can be so profound and so healing. Music allows you to experience your feelings that get ignored and suppressed in daily life. Music allows you to experience the feelings that are buried inside of you. This is the healing power of music—the profound ability of musical notes to unearth feelings of loss and sadness that you haven't experienced in a long time and find comfort in this process.

This discovering of long buried away feelings can help you heal just like removing a splinter from a finger. Have you ever had a splinter in your finger that was there for days or weeks or even longer? Some days you may not even feel it, but other days it causes irritation and pain. Repressed emotional pain from the past is sort of like that. It can be buried deep inside of you and doesn't seem to cause any problems for a long period of time. However, the pain is still there and one day it will begin to damage your health unless you deal with it effectively.

I'm sure you may have your own personal story of how music found a way into your heart during a particularly difficult time. Patients often ask which types of music provide the most healing benefits and that depends on the individual. Find the genre of music that touches you in a meaningful way whether it's classical, folk, rock, jazz, reggae, electronic, pop, hip-hop, or country. Find the type of music that helps you get in touch with your feelings, whether they're feelings of joy or sadness. Music can help bring you tremendous joy and it can also help heal the wounds that you may still be carrying from the past.

Just like a tweezer removing that splinter, music can be a tool to cut through your psychological barriers to reach deep inside and unearth unresolved and unprocessed emotional pain. There are numerous studies from the last decade that show that music offers many healing benefits. Make music a part of your life if it isn't already. Enjoy it, savor it, and allow it to reach the depths of who you are and help you heal whatever pain lies deep inside.

Michael is a 51 year old writer who came to see me because of a rash on his abdomen. He originally thought that it might be poison ivy because he had gone hiking last weekend, but over-the-counter hydrocortisone cream didn't help much. He didn't recall having this sort of rash before. I took a look at Michael's rash and it looked like a small clusters of blisters, which is the classic appearance of shingles. Michael and I discussed the diagnosis and I prescribed medication.

Because shingles tends to occur during times of high stress, I asked if he had recently experienced any difficult situations. After a long pause, Michael told me that he lost his sister a couple of months ago after a long battle with brain cancer. The loss had been devastating to Michael. To cope with the loss, Michael said he's been eating a lot more and drinking a lot of wine.

I told Michael that I was concerned about him drinking this much alcohol. I asked him if there might be other ways for him to spend his time. The topic of music came up because Michael had just seen one of his favorite bands in concert that week. As we discussed music, Michael's mood perked up. He told me that was quite the guitarist back in his teenage years. In fact, his sister played piano and they used to play music together in their family's garage. Though his dream of starting a rock band with his sister never materialized, Michael told me that music has remained a major part of his life.

After our visit, Michael created a website to honor his sister and included several touching music videos in her memory. Michael then decided to use the website to raise money for several cancer charities. Michael also told me that he's returned to playing the guitar and is recording an album. That was his childhood dream and he told me that the loss of his sister had inspired him to make every moment count, whether it's at work or in his personal life. Michael then told me that he learned that the best way for him to move forward after this major loss is to carry on his sister's life in everything he does. He said that, in some small way, his sister can live on in his music.

❖ ❖ ❖

Habit 49: Forgiveness

In habit 42, we discussed the importance of letting go of emotional pain related to past experiences. In this habit, we will discuss the importance of letting go of the grievances that we have against others. This process is called forgiveness.

Have you ever met someone who is still angry at someone over something that happened years ago? It could be someone who can't move on from what someone did to them in the past. It could be someone who is still actively estranged from a loved one because of something that is ancient history. Holding grudges for many years is more common than you'd think. Perhaps you know someone who's in this category. If so, it's important to recognize that there's a health benefit to finding forgiveness and letting go of past grievances and regrets. Of all the habits of *The Wellness Code*, this is one of the most challenging and most rewarding.

When I say that you should let go of past grievances, that doesn't mean that you should pretend that the past didn't happen or ignore what people have done in the past. That would be foolish.

Letting go of past grievances means that you end the emotional power that the past has over your current life. You disconnect what happened in the past from how you feel today. This is what is meant by true forgiveness. Forgiveness means accepting your past and neutralizing the emotional power it has over your present life. Forgiveness does not always mean that you necessarily restore a relationship with the person who wronged you. Moreover, forgiveness does not mean that you condone what happened in the past. It simply means that what happened in the past no longer has a physical or emotional impact on you.

For example, many adult victims of child abuse find it freeing to forgive their parents. By doing so, they get to the point where the abuse no longer has an effect on how they function today. However, this doesn't necessarily mean that they reestablish a relationship with their parents and pretend that nothing happened.

Forgiveness is an internal process. You still remember what happened in the past, but your current emotional state is no longer affected. Often in situations like this, the person doing the forgiving does so in the context of going through therapy and never communicates their forgiveness to the transgressor. The forgiveness isn't intended to make the perpetrator feel better or to restore any relationship. The relationship may be restored, but that is not necessarily related to the forgiveness itself. The status of the relationship with the parent is separate from the forgiveness process. It's possible to reestablish a relationship with someone you've forgiven and it's also possible to not do so.

In your life, you may have situations from the past where you've been hurt and there may be people that you need to forgive. If you have situations like this, remember that forgiveness is really about helping yourself move on from the past rather than helping the transgressor. In such cases, forgiveness is intended to help you accept and move on from the reality of the past and lessen the impact the past event has on your present life.

This was one of the lessons that my Grandma Emma tried to teach me when I was a child. She must have told me at least once a month, "When you forgive someone, you free someone from prison and you realize that the prisoner is you." Grandma Emma realized that the true beneficiary of forgiveness is the person doing the forgiving.

There are several ideas that can help with the forgiveness process. First, as we have discussed, realize what forgiveness is—it's letting go of the control that the past has over you. It has little to do with the transgressor. You forgive to free yourself from the past, not to let the other person off the hook. You accept that the past happened and you decide that it won't affect how you feel or act anymore.

Second, you realize that, in all likelihood, the person did not intentionally try to hurt you. It may seem like they did, but in most cases the person did whatever they did because of their own issues. Most likely, it was a way to meet their own needs and deal with pain that they "inherited" or learned from prior generations. In all likelihood, hurting you was an unintended consequence of them acting out their own issues. Realizing this can help to begin the process of releasing a grievance.

The final part of the process is to approach forgiveness from the opposite perspective. Find a situation in your life where you hurt someone else and contact them and apologize for what you did. It may be something really small, such as being short tempered with someone at the office. It could be something more significant. Whether big or small, admitting and apologizing for your own past transgressions helps you to begin to heal the pain and anger associated with your grievances against others. It works. By apologizing to others, you gain an appreciation of another perspective and it becomes easier to forgive. Forgiveness works to release you from the past and stop the cycle of emotional pain from ancient hurts. This frees you to live fully in the present and get the most out of each moment of your life.

◆ ◆ ◆

Stacy is a 29 year old patient of mine who's a graduate student at a major university. She came to see me because her boyfriend was concerned about her drinking and her poor sleep habits. She told me about his concerns and she also told me that one of her deepest fears is that she will become an alcoholic. I asked her where this fear came from and she said that her mother was an alcoholic who died in a car crash when Stacy was only five years old. Stacy doesn't remember much about her mother but she told me that she's always been angry at her mother for driving while intoxicated and leaving her to be raised by a single father.

Stacy also told me about her own struggles with anxiety, which have been a lifelong issue for her. She noticed in high school that when she drank alcohol, all of her anxieties and fears drifted away and she felt liberated and free to be herself. For her, alcohol was a way of soothing the anxiety that she has lived with for years. We talked about all of this and I could see light bulbs starting to go off in her head. She was starting to see the connections between her mother's life and death and her own struggles.

I asked Stacy to think about two things. First, we discussed that everyone makes mistakes; that we all say or do things that we will regret. In her mother's case, sadly, the decision to drive while drunk cost her life. I asked Stacy to think about her mom who died at about the same age that she is right now. I asked her to assume that her mother probably had the same proclivity toward alcohol that she does, and to try to put herself in her mother's shoes and realize that we can all make mistakes.

And secondly, and most importantly, I asked her to think about forgiveness and consider forgiving her mother even though she has passed. I explained to her that when you forgive, you let go of the pain and anger associated with the past. You don't necessarily agree with or condone what happened but you accept the fact that it happened and let go of your feelings about it. When you hold on to grievances, anger and resentment, you are figuratively keeping yourself in the prison of your painful past.

In Stacy's case, she was still holding on to her anger against her mother. The anxiety, sleep issues, and alcohol abuse resulted from holding on to these feelings, and this was damaging Stacy's life. This lack of forgiveness was clearly impacting her health, happiness, and possibly her longevity. Stacy and I had a productive office visit and she said that she would think a lot about everything we discussed, including attending an AA meeting which was something her boyfriend had also suggested. She left my office that afternoon with the beginnings of a plan for what will hopefully become a new way of life for her.

❖ ❖ ❖

During your life, you will revisit thoughts, feelings, and experiences many times. Because life often feels like a circle, it is easy to fall into the trap of believing that your life is all about the past and the future. In fact, your life is really about the present moment. You can learn from your past and plan for your future, but you only truly live life in each moment. If too much of your time is spent focused on negatives from the past or possible problems in the future, it is difficult to enjoy each precious moment of life.

Every time you start focusing on a grievance that you have with someone, try to find a way to practice forgiveness. The more that you can release your past grievances and move on from that past pain, the healthier you will be both emotionally and physically. The toll of carrying anger and resentment is very significant, so be sure to practice forgiveness whenever possible.

Think through situations that happened in your past that you believe are negatively impacting your life today. Whether you choose to speak directly with the person who has hurt you, journal privately about the situation, or discuss the situation with a third party, search your heart to find forgiveness and free yourself from the past.

To live in the present, you must free yourself from the effects of the past.

Habit 50: Practice Mindfulness

In habit 20, I discussed the power of meditation and the effects it can have on your peace of mind and your happiness. With meditation, you learn to focus your attention on the present moment whether it's through the use of a prayer, mantra, or movement. Having a consistent meditation practice can provide tremendous benefits to how you feel, as well as your health, happiness, and longevity. Meditation is usually something that is practiced for short periods of time. What would happen if you expanded the practice of meditation so that you focus your attention on the present moment through the entire day? That's the practice of mindfulness.

Mindfulness has been defined in many different ways over the years. There is the practice of mindfulness meditation, which is a specific type of meditation practice. My definition of mindfulness is the practice of staying connected to the present moment throughout every moment of your day. In practical terms, this means paying attention to what you are doing with every breath, every thought, and every movement. It means that you notice people, places, and things that you see and avoid living life on cruise control.

In this sense, mindfulness is the extension of meditation into your entire life. It means you focus your attention on the present moment— not the past or future—at all times. By doing so, you stay engaged in life with your focus on what's happening to you right now.

This can seem daunting at first, but mindfulness is profoundly healing and nourishing to the body, mind, and spirit.

There are many tools and strategies that can help you stay rooted in the present moment. Periodically feeling the breath enter and leave your lungs is one way. Remembering to notice other people and aspects of your environment is also very helpful. For example, make it a habit to consciously make at least five observations about every place that you go. For example, if you go to a restaurant, you might notice a song being played, the name of the waiter, your favorite part of the meal, the name of the restaurant, and a piece of art hanging on the wall. One of the keys to mindfulness is to constantly notice your environment.

Another helpful tool to bring you back to the present moment is to practice, "This is the only time." It is simple, but it works wonders. As you go through your day, savor each and every moment because moments come and go and aren't repeated. This concept was powerfully depicted in the series finale of the television show *Six Feet Under* when Nate says to his sister Claire, "You can't take a picture of this, it's already gone."

Do your best to stay focused on the current moment. Stay focused on the person with whom you're speaking. Stay focused on the movie you're watching or the article you're reading. Stay focused on your kids, your spouse, or your parents. Stay focused on everyone with whom you spend time. Stay fully engaged and fully present in each moment of your life.

However, you are human and at times your mind will drift. Your thoughts will drift into the past or into the future and away from the present moment. When this happens, one of the best tools to bring you back to the present moment is to remind yourself that this exact moment will never happen again. It can be a sad thought, but you will never have this exact moment again. You may have similar moments in the future, but you will never have this exact moment ever again.

For example, let's say you're attending your daughter's third grade school play and you find yourself losing focus on the moment. You want to enjoy every moment of the play, but you keep thinking about a work project. As soon as you find your mind drifting away from the present moment, remind yourself that this is the only time you will ever have this exact experience again. Realizing this has a tremendous power to bring you back into the present moment.

Let's say it is your son's graduation from college and you find yourself zoning out during the long commencement speech. You start thinking about work or a big football game. When you find your thoughts drifting away, remind yourself that this is the only time you will attend your son's college graduation.

Even on a seemingly ordinary day, remind yourself that this is the only time you will have this specific day ever again. Reminders like this help you to enjoy the day and savor the experience before it becomes a memory.

Sometimes I get a lump in my throat just thinking in these terms. This feeling is a powerful tool to center you and bring you back to the present moment. It helps to break the chain of worries about the future or concerns about the past. It re-engages you in the now. It is easy to get distracted and fall into the trap that something else is more important than fully experiencing this current moment. However, if you lose touch with the present moment, you become an observer of life instead of an active participant.

Be an active participant in your life by using mindfulness tools. As you go through your day, keep reminding yourself, "This is the only time." Find other tools to help bring your attention back to the present moment. Use the practice of making five different observations everywhere you go. Use your breath to center yourself and keep you rooted in the now. See what practices work for you. The goal is to enjoy and savor every moment of your life. This is the core practice of mindfulness or full engagement in life.

Start by practicing this for an hour a day. Spend an hour each day fully present in what you're doing. Don't think about your emails or how long it's been since you posted something online. Pay full attention to the conversation you're having, the meal you're eating, the movie you're watching, or the music you're hearing. Be fully mindful and present in your life.

CHAPTER 7:

Conclusion:
Living The Wellness Code

Congratulations! You've reached the end of this book, which is a great accomplishment and means that you are serious about creating a life of wellness. While this is the end of the book, it is just the beginning of your healthier approach to life. Your next step is to start implementing *The Wellness Code* and integrating the habits into your lifestyle.

I recommend that you start with the four column process as detailed in chapter 9, which will help you self-evaluate and prioritize your habits each month. The four column exercise is the entry point to living *The Wellness Code* and the key to making this program come to life. Review all fifty habits and sort the habits into the four columns, and then pick your two habits for the first month. Have fun with the habits. This is the adventure that is your life. Make it an amazing month as you strive to make these two new habits a consistent part of who you are and how you live. Your goal is to integrate these two new habits into your life. Do the very best you can, but be kind to yourself. If you're less than successful one day, get up the next morning and try again.

At the end of each month, make an honest assessment of how things went. What went well? What didn't? Did these two new habits become a part of your life? After you've made this assessment, go back and re-do the four column process for the next month. With fresh eyes, take another look at all fifty habits and place them in their correct columns. Make sure that the habits in column one still belong there. Make sure the habits in column two really belong there, and so on.

Then, choose your two habits for the next month. They can be the same two habits from the prior month if those habits aren't yet in column one. If you feel that you're better equipped to try another habit, then go for that. Either way, choose your two habits for the next month from column two.

You'll be repeating this process every month going forward as you gradually shift your habits towards wellness. On a quarterly basis, I recommend that you do a more comprehensive evaluation of your progress. These quarterly evaluations are an ideal time to think about the habits in columns three and four. Read about the habits in column four to see if something resonates with you and triggers a movement to column three. Do the same with the habits in column three. For each habit that's not in column one, make a list of why you should and why you shouldn't practice each one. Also, list all the roadblocks to accomplishing each habit and think about what you could do to remove these hurdles. Is it a scheduling issue? Is it a situational issue? Perhaps your life has changed to the point where some of the habits in column three could be moved to column two. The goal, for now, is to move as many habits as possible towards column two as those are the habits which can be considered to be actively practiced each month. Sometimes it's easy to focus on the habits in column two, but don't forget to put work into the habits in the third and fourth columns. That's the work that happens each quarter. This sort of work takes time, but you will find that previously unappealing habits start to seem doable as they make their way to the left side of the chart.

On an annual basis, I recommend that you step back and take a look at how you've done for the year. Congratulate yourself for all of your accomplishments. Notice the habits that you're now practicing on a consistent basis. That's great work! During these annual reviews, I recommend that you enlist someone else to review the columns with you. This person should be someone who knows you well: perhaps a close family member or friend. With this person's help, review all of the habits with a focus on better understanding what is holding back the habits that aren't in column one. In particular, notice the habits that have moved from column three to column two. Notice the habits that have moved from column four to column three, which is a big deal. Habits in column three are now close to being considered for your monthly habits. Your healthier lifestyle is reflected in the number of habits that have shifted to the left.

Also, notice the habits that have slipped back and moved to the right of the table as well as the habits that haven't shifted. Don't get down on yourself. Realize that this is very tough life-changing work and this takes time and patience. You're in this for the long-term and there will be bumps in the road to wellness.

A healthy lifestyle doesn't happen overnight. *The Wellness Code* is not quick-fix diet or program. Rather it is a long-term process where you gradually move forward into wellness—into a life of optimal health, happiness, and longevity. During your annual evaluation, I also recommend that you meet with a mentor with whom you can discuss how you did for the year. Your mentor should be someone who can give you positive feedback and encouragement on your successes, but also who is comfortable discussing the habits in depth. It's often helpful to review your struggles with your mentor and brainstorm ideas for the upcoming year. More than anything, your mentor should be someone who helps keep you accountable and focused on practicing a healthier lifestyle.

Enjoy the process. Remember to smile. Make it fun and savor your experiences. As you continue to practice this process day after day and month after month, be sure to share this information with others. Pass this information forward. Teach the principles of *The Wellness Code* to someone who might be in need. As you continue to practice the process, my hope is that, in addition to finding improved health and longevity, you will also find greater satisfaction and fulfillment in your life. Remember the three goals of *The Wellness Code*: longevity, health, and happiness. These three interdependent goals are wellsprings that can be passed onto your friends, family, and future generations.

I sincerely hope that this book has helped and will continue to help you. I always enjoy hearing from those who are practicing *The Wellness Code* so please let me know how the book has impacted your life. You can reach me at drmorris@drbrianmorris.com or check out my website www.drbrianmorris.com for updates on future projects. It's been a privilege and an honor to have this opportunity to share *The Wellness Code* with you. I hope this information continues to inspire and guide you on your journey to optimal wellness.

Acknowledgements

First and foremost, I'd like to thank my wife Rebecca, who is my partner in this adventure of life. You have been, and will always be, the love of my life and the best role model that our children could ever have. The suggestions and edits that you made added so much to this book. I'd also like to thank our four amazing children who inspire me every day to be a better father and human being.

I'd like to thank my extended family, including my father Dr. Stephen Morris, my mother Judith Morris, my father-in-law Joseph Tuchinsky, my mother-in-law Cele Tuchinsky, my brother Kevin Morris, my sister-in-law Wendy Morris, my uncle Chuck Morris, my aunt Becky Morris, and cousins Brittney Morris Saunders, Tim Saunders, Kolby Morris, Isabel Morris, Sophie Morris, Zachary Morris, Lincoln Saunders, and Sadie Morris. I am fortunate to be surrounded by such a loving and supportive family. I also want to thank my late grandparents Emma Morris, Fred Morris, Ruth Teichman, and Morris Teichman for always believing in me.

I'd like to thank Dr. Arvind Prabhat for the thirty years of friendship that started in that calculus class at University of Pennsylvania. Thank you for all of your encouragement and unwavering support.

Thank you to my medical colleagues and our amazing team at The UCLA Comprehensive Health Program who always prioritize the care and well-being of our patients. Specifically, thank you to Cyrus Baraghoush, Julie Escobar, Alex Godoy, Patricia Hurtado, Julia Kaminer, Abigail Katsen, Natalie Kodikian, Zoua Lee, Claudia Marin, Gladys Martinez, Wendy Pitts, Brittany Uy, Jeanette Villegas, Keisha Warren, Dr. Ben Ansell, Dr. Karen Cheng, and Dr. Camelia Davtyan.

I'd also like to thank each and every patient that I've seen over the last twenty plus years. You've given me the privilege to practice the art of medicine, which is the joy of my professional life. I'm also grateful to past and present colleagues who helped shape my professional life including Dr. Phil Triffletti, Dr. Martin True, Dr. Lyle Kaliser, and Dr. Ben Ansell. I'd also like to thank the medical students and housestaff whom I've trained at Harvard and UCLA. You have taught me just as much as I hope I've taught you.

Scientific Reference Articles and Suggested Readings

Introduction and Chapter 1

"Amok Time." *Star Trek*. NBC. September 15, 1967. Television.

Jerry Maguire. Dir Cameron Crowe. 1996. Sony Pictures Home Entertainment. DVD.

Chapter 2

Campbell J, *The Hero With A Thousand Faces*. Novato, California: New World Library, 2008.

Mann T, Tomiyama AJ, Westling E, Lew AM, Samuels B, Chatman J, "Medicare's search for effective obesity treatments: diets are not the answer," *Am Psychol*. 2007 Apr;62(3):220-33.

Fildes A, Charlton J, Rudisill C, Littlejohns P, Prevost AT, Gulliford MC, "Probability of an Obese Person Attaining Normal Body Weight: Cohort Study Using Electronic Health Records," *Am J Public Health*. 2015 Sep;105(9):e54-9.

Benson H, Stark M, *Timeless Healing: The Power and Biology of Belief*. New York, New York: Simon & Schuster, 1996.

Chapter 3

Ludovici AM, *Change Your Mind, Change Your Health: 7 Ways to Harness the Power of Your Brain to Achieve True Well-Being*. Pompton Plains, New Jersey: New Page Books, 2014.

Meyers, D. G, *Social Psychology (11th Ed)*. New York, New York: McGraw- Hill, 2012.

Covey, SR, Merrill, RA, Merrill, RR, *First Things First: To Live, To Learn, to Leave a Legacy*. New York, New York: Simon & Schuster, 1994.

Prochaska JO, Norcross JC, Diclemente CC, *Changing For Good: A Revolutionary Six-Stage Program For Overcoming Bad Habits and Moving Your Life Positively Forward*. New York, New York: Harper Collins, 1994.

Chapter 4

Ludovici AM, *Change Your Mind, Change Your Health: 7 Ways to Harness the Power of Your*

Brain to Achieve True Well-Being. Pompton Plains, New Jersey: New Page Books, 2014.

Prochaska JO, Norcross JC, Diclemente CC, *Changing For Good: A Revolutionary Six-Stage Program For Overcoming Bad Habits and Moving Your Life Positively Forward*. New York, New York: Harper Collins, 1994.

Vogler C, *Mythic Structures For Writers*. Studio City, California: Michael Wiese Productions, 2008.

Covey SR, *The 7 Habits of Highly Effective People*. New York, New York: Simon & Schuster, 1989.

Chapter 5

Mueller PA, Oppenheimer DM, "The pen is mightier than the keyboard: advantages of longhand over laptop note taking," *Psychol Sci*. 2014 Jun;25(6):1159-68.

Meyers, D. G, *Social Psychology (11th Ed)*. New York, New York: McGraw- Hill, 2012.

Chapter 6

Nutrition

Habit 1: Eat the Correct Number of Calories

Sacks FM, Bray GA, "Carey VJ, et al. Comparison of weight-loss diets with different compositions of fat, protein, and carbohydrates," *N Engl J Med*. 2009;360:859-873.

Gardner, CD, et al, "Comparison of the Atkins, Zone, Ornish, and LEARN diets for change in weight and related risk factors among overweight premenopausal women: the A TO Z Weight Loss Study: a randomized trial," *JAMA*. 2007;297(9):969-77.

Bacigalupo R, Cudd P, Littlewood C, Bissell P, Hawley MS, Buckley Woods H, "Interventions employing mobile technology for overweight and obesity: an early systematic review of randomized controlled trials," *Obes Rev*. 2013;14(4):279–291.

Burke LE, Wang J, Sevick MA, "Self-monitoring in weight loss: a systematic review of the literature," *J Am Diet Assoc*. 2011;111(1):92–102.

Helsel DL, Jakicic JM, Otto AD, "Comparison of techniques for self-monitoring eating and exercise behaviors on weight loss in a correspondence-based intervention," *J Am Diet Assoc*. 2007;107(10):1807–1810.

Cadmus-Bertram L, Wang JB, Patterson RE, Newman VA, Parker BA, Pierce JP, "Web-based self-monitoring for weight loss among overweight/obese women at increased risk for breast cancer: the HELP pilot study," *Psychooncology*. 2013 Aug;22(8):1821-8.

Teague C, O'Connor A, *Lose It!: The Personalized Weight Loss Revolution*. Emmaus, Pennsylvania: Rodale Books, 2010.

Burke LE, Conroy MB, Sereika SM, et al, "The effect of electronic self-monitoring on weight loss and dietary intake: a randomized behavioral weight loss trial," *Obesity*. 2011;19(2):338–344.

Freedman MR, King J, Kennedy E, "Popular diets: a scientific review," *Obes Res*. 2001;9:(Suppl):1S-40S.

Brehm BJ, Seeley RJ, Daniels SR, D'Alessio DA, "A randomized trial comparing a very low carbohydrate diet and a calorie-restricted low fat diet on body weight and cardiovascular risk factors in healthy women," *J Clin Endocrinol Metab.* 2003;88:1617-1623.

Foster GD, Wyatt HR, Hill JO, et al, "A randomized trial of a low-carbohydrate diet for obesity," *N Engl J Med.* 2003;348:2082-2090.

Samaha FF, Iqbal N, Seshadri P, et al, "A low-carbohydrate as compared with a low-fat diet in severe obesity," *N Engl J Med.* 2003;348:2074-2081.

Yancy WS Jr, Olsen MK, Guyton JR, Bakst RP, Westman EC, "A low-carbohydrate ketogenic diet versus a low-fat diet to treat obesity and hyperlipidemia: a randomized, controlled trial," *Ann Intern Med.* 2004;140:769-777.

Due A, Toubro S, Skov AR, Astrup A, "Effect of normal-fat diets, either medium or high in protein, on body weight in overweight subjects: a randomised 1-year trial," *Int J Obes Relat Metab Disord.* 2004;28:1283-1290.

Habit 2: Eat the Correct Types of Calories

Ebbeling CB, Swain JF, Feldman HA, et al, "Effects of Dietary Composition on Energy Expenditure During Weight-Loss Maintenance," *JAMA.* 2012;307(24):2627-2634.

Mozaffarian D, Hao T, Rimm EB, Willett WC, Hu FB, "Changes in diet and lifestyle and long-term weight gain in women and men," *N Engl J Med.* 2011 Jun 23;364(25):2392-404.

Larsen, T.M., et al "Diets with high or low protein content and glycemic index for weight-loss maintenance," *N Engl J Med,* 2010. 363(22): 2102-13.

Ornish, D, *The Spectrum: A Scientifically Proven Program to Feel Better, Live Longer, Lose Weight, and Gain Health.* New York, New York: Ballantine Books, 2008.

Heber D, Bowerman S, *What Color Is Your Diet?* New York, New York: Harper Collins, 2001.

Rolls B, Hermann M, *The Ultimate Volumetrics Diet: Smart, Simple, Science-Based Strategies For Losing Weight and Keeping It Off.* New York, New York: Harper Collins, 2012.

Rahman K, "Studies on free radicals, antioxidants, and co-factors," *Clin Interv Aging.* 2007 Jun; 2(2): 219–236.

Mayo Clinic Staff, "Supplements: Nutrition in a pill?" *MayoClinic.com.* October 18, 2014.

Kloner RA, Rezkalla SH, "To drink or not to drink? That is the question," *Circulation.* 2007; 116:1306–17.

Nanney MS, Haire-Joshu D, Hessler K, Brownson RC, "Rationale for a consistent "powerhouse" approach to vegetable and fruit messages," *J Am Diet Assoc.* 2004;104(3):352–6.

Campbell MK, Carr C, Devellis B, Switzer B, Biddle A, Amamoo M.A, "A randomized trial of tailoring and motivational interviewing to promote fruit and vegetable consumption for cancer prevention and control," *Ann Behav Med.* 2009;38:71–85.

Kulie T, Groff A, Redmer J, Hounshell J, Schrager S, "Vitamin D: an evidence-based review," *J Am Board Fam Med.* 2009 Nov-Dec;22(6):698-706.

Campbell MK, Carr C, Devellis B, Switzer B, Biddle A, Amamoo M.A, "A randomized trial of tailoring and motivational interviewing to promote fruit and vegetable consumption for cancer prevention and control," *Ann Behav Med.* 2009;38:71–85.

Higdon JV, Delage B, Williams DE, Dashwood RH, "Cruciferous vegetables and human cancer risk: epidemiologic evidence and mechanistic basis," *Pharmacol Res.* 2007;55(3):224–36.

Dietary Guidelines Advisory Committee, "Report of the Dietary Guidelines Advisory Committee on the Dietary Guidelines for Americans, 2010, to the Secretary of Agriculture and the Secretary of Health and Human Services." Washington (DC): US Department of Agriculture, Agricultural Research Service; 2010.

Darmon N, Darmon M, Maillot M, Drewnowski A, "A nutrient density standard for vegetables and fruits: nutrients per calorie and nutrients per unit cost." *J Am Diet Assoc.* 2005;105(12):1881–7.

Otten JJ, Hellwig JP, Meyers LD, editors, *Dietary reference intakes: the essential guide to nutrient requirements*, Washington, D.C.: National Academies Press, 2006.

Habit 3: Downsize Your Eating Habits

Wansink B, *Mindless Eating: Why We Eat More Than We Think*, New York, New York: Random House, 2006.

Fletcher AM, *Thin For Life: 10 Keys To Success From People Who Have Lost Weight And Kept It Off*, New York, New York: Houghton Mifflin Company, 2003.

Squires S, *Secrets of The Lean Plate Club: A Simple, Step-By-Step Program To Help You Shed Pounds and Keep Them Off For Good*, New York, New York: St. Martin's Press, 2006.

Wansink B, Shimizu M, Cardello AV, Wright AO, *Dining in the Dark: How Uncertainty Influences Food Acceptance in the Dark. Food Quality and Preference*, 2012;24:1:209-212.

Chandon P, Wansink B, "Is Food Marketing Making Us Fat? A Multi-Disciplinary Review," *Foundations and Trends in Marketing.* 2011;5:3:113-196.

Payne CR, Wansink B, "Quantitative Approaches to Consumer Field Research," *Journal of Marketing Theory and Practice.* 2011;19:4:377-389.

Shimizu M, Wansink B, "Watching Food-related Television Increases Caloric Intake in Restrained Eaters," *Appetite.* 2011;57:661-664.

Just DR, Wansink B, "The Flat-rate Pricing Paradox: Conflicting Effects of 'All-You-Can-Eat' Buffet Pricing," *The Review of Economics and Statistics.* 2011;93:193-200.

Scheibehenne B, Todd PM, Wansink B, "Dining in the Dark: The Importance of Visual Cues for Food Consumption and Satiety," *Appetite.* 2010;55:3:710-713.

Wansink B, Painter JE, Lee YK, "The office candy dish: proximity's influence on estimated and actual consumption," *Int J Obes (Lond).* 2006 May;30(5):871-5.

Shimizu M, Payne CR, Wansink B, "When snacks become meals: how hunger and environmental cues bias food intake," *International Journal of Behavioral Nutrition and Physical Activity.* 2010;7:63:25.

Habit 4: The ADAPT Process

Downie C, *The Spark: The 28-Day Breakthrough Plan for Losing Weight, Getting Fit, and Transforming Your Life*, Carlsbad, California: Hay House, 2009.

Wing RR, Phelan S, "Long-term weight loss maintenance," *Am J Clin Nutr.* 2005;82(Suppl):222S–225S.

Teague C, O'Connor A, *Lose It!: The Personalized Weight Loss Revolution*, Emmaus, Pennsylvania: Rodale Books, 2010.

Shilts MK, Horowitz M, Townsend MS, "Goal setting as a strategy for dietary and physical activity behavior change: a review of the literature," *Am J Health Promot.* 2004;19(2):81–93.

Astrup A., Rossner S, "Lessons from obesity management programmes: greater initial weight loss improves long-term maintenance," *Obesity Reviews.* 2000;1(1):17–19.

Streit KJ. Stevens NH. Stevens VJ. Rossner J, "Food records: a predictor and modifier of weight change in a long-term weight loss program." *J Am Diet Assoc.* 1991;91:213–216.

Tsai AG, Wadden TA, "Systematic review: an evaluation of major commercial weight loss programs in the United States," *Annals of Internal Medicine.* 2005;142(1):56–66.

Elfhag K., Rossner S, "Who succeeds in maintaining weight loss? A conceptual review of factors associated with weight loss maintenance and weight regain," *Obesity Reviews.* 2005;6(1):67–85.

Sherwood NE, Crain AL, Martinson BC, et al, "Enhancing long-term weight loss maintenance: 2-year results from the Keep It Off randomized controlled trial," *Preventive Medicine.* 2013;56(3-4):171–177.

Perri MG, Limacher MC, Durning PE, et al, "Extended-care programs for weight management in rural communities: the treatment of obesity in underserved rural settings (TOURS) randomized trial," *Archives of Internal Medicine,* 2008;168(21):2347–2354.

Cussler EC, Teixeira PJ, Going SB, et al, "Maintenance of weight loss in overweight middle-aged women through the internet," *Obesity.* 2008;16(5):1052–1060.

Harvey-Berino J, Pintauro S, Buzzell P, Gold EC, "Effect of internet support on the long-term maintenance of weight loss," *Obesity Research.* 2004;12(2):320–329.

Stevens VJ, Obarzanek E, Cook NR, et al, "Long-term weight loss and changes in blood pressure: results of the trials of hypertension prevention, phase II," *Annals of Internal Medicine.* 2001;134(1):1–11.

Pearson ES, "Goal setting as a health behavior change strategy in overweight and obese adults: a systematic literature review examining intervention components," *Patient Educ Couns.* 2012 Apr;87(1):32-42.

Habit 5: Eat Before You Eat

Flood-Obbagy JE, Rolls BJ, "The effect of fruit in different forms on energy intake and satiety at a meal," *Appetite.* 2009 Apr;52(2):416-22.

Hetherington MM, Regan MF, "Effects of chewing gum on short-term appetite regulation in moderately restrained eaters," *Appetite.* 2011 Oct;57(2):475-82.

Higgs S, Jones A, "Prolonged chewing at lunch decreases later snack intake," *Appetite.* 2013 Mar;62:91-5.

Almiron-Roig E, Flores SY, Drewnowski A, "No difference in satiety or in subsequent energy intakes between a beverage and a solid food," *Physiology and Behavior.* 2004;82:671–677.

Flood JE, Rolls BJ, Roe LS, "The effect of increased beverage portion size on energy intake at a meal," *Journal of the American Dietetic Association.* 2006;106:1984–1990.

Flood J, Rolls B, "Soup preloads in a variety of forms reduce meal energy intake," *Appetite.* 2007;49:626–634.

Howarth NC, Saltzman E, Roberts SB, "Dietary fiber and weight regulation," *Nutrition Reviews.* 2001;59:129–139.

Mattes R, "Soup and satiety," *Physiology and Behavior.* 2005;83:739–747.

Rolls BJ, Fedoroff IC, Guthrie JF, Laster LJ, "Foods with different satiating effects in humans," *Appetite.* 1990 Oct;15(2):115-26.

Rolls BJ, Drewnowski A, Ledikwe JH, "Changing the energy density of the diet as a strategy for weight management," *Journal of the American Dietetic Association.* 2005;10:S98–S103.

Habit 6: Make Healthy Food Convenient

Gilhooly CH, Das SK, Golden JK, et al, "Food cravings and energy regulation: the characteristics of craved foods and their relationship with eating behaviors and weight change during 6 months of dietary energy restriction," *International Journal of Obesity.* 2007;31(12):1849–1858.

Wansink B, Painter JE, Lee YK, "The office candy dish: proximity's influence on estimated and actual consumption," *Int J Obes.* 2006 May;30(5):871-5.

Glanz K, Basil M, Maibach E, Goldberg J, Snyder D, "Why Americans eat what they do: taste, nutrition, cost, convenience, and weight control concerns as influences on food consumption," *J Am Diet Assoc.* 1998;98:1118–1126. |

Sporny LA, Contento IR, "Stages of change in dietary fat reduction social psychological correlates," *J Nutr Educ.* 1995;27:191–199.

Patel KA, Schlundt DG, "Impact of moods and social context on eating behavior," *Appetite.* 2001; 36: 111–118.

Oliver G, Wardle J, Gibson L, "Stress, food choice: a laboratory study," *Psychosomatic Med.* 2000; 62: 853–865.

Berry SL, Beatty WW, Klesges RC, "Sensory, social influences on ice cream consumption by males, females in a laboratory setting," *Appetite.* 1985;6:41–45.

Terry K, Beck S, "Eating style, food storage habits in the home: Assessment of obese, non-obese families," *Behav Modification.* 1985;9:242–261.

Painter JE, Wansink B, Hieggelke JB, "How visibility, convenience influence candy consumption," *Appetite.* 2002;38:237–238.

Chandon P, Wansink B, "Does stockpiling accelerate consumption. A convenience-salience framework of consumption stockpiling," *J Marketing Res.* 2002;39:321–335.

Levitsky DA, "Putting behavior back into feeding behavior: a tribute to George Collier," *Appetite.* 2002;38:143–148.

Wansink B, Cheney MM, "Super bowls: serving bowl size and food consumption," *JAMA.* 2005;293:1727–1728.

Habit 7: Eat Breakfast

Elfhag K, Rossner S, "Who succeeds in maintaining weight loss? A conceptual review of factors associated with weight loss maintenance and weight regain," *Obes Rev.* 2005;6(1):67–85.

Deshmukh-Taskar PR1, Nicklas TA, O'Neil CE, Keast DR, Radcliffe JD, Cho S, "The relationship of breakfast skipping and type of breakfast consumption with nutrient intake and weight status in children and adolescents: the National Health and Nutrition Examination Survey 1999-2006," *J Am Diet Assoc.* 2010 Jun;110(6):869-78.

Kochar J, Djousse L, Gaziano JM, "Breakfast cereals and risk of type 2 diabetes in the Physicians' Health Study I," *Obesity* (Silver Spring) 2007;15:3039-3044.

Liu S, Sesso HD, Manson JE, Willett WC, Buring JE, "Is intake of breakfast cereals related to total and cause-specific mortality in men?" *Am J Clin Nutr* 2003;77:594-599.

Bazzano LA, Song Y, Bubes V, Good CK, Manson JE, Liu S, "Dietary intake of whole and refined grain breakfast cereals and weight gain in men," *Obes Res.* 2005;13:1952-1960.

De la Hunty A, Ashwell M, "Are people who regularly eat breakfast cereals slimmer than those who don't? A systematic review of the evidence," *Nutr Bull.* 2007;32:118-128.

Rampersaud GC, Pereira MA, Girard BL, Adams J, Metzl JD, "Breakfast habits, nutritional status, body weight, and academic performance in children and adolescents," *J Am Diet Assoc.* 2005;105:743-760.

Kosti RI, Panagiotakos DB, Zampelas A, "Ready-to-eat cereals and the burden of obesity in the context of their nutritional contribution: are all ready-to-eat cereals equally healthy? A systematic review," *Nutr Res Rev.* 2010;23:314-322.

McNulty H, Eaton-Evans J, Cran G, Woulahan G, Boreham C, Savage JM, Fletcher R, Strain JJ, "Nutrient intakes and impact of fortified breakfast cereals in schoolchildren," *Arch Dis Child.* 1996;75:474-481.

Timlin MT, Pereira MA, Story M, Neumark-Sztainer D, "Breakfast eating and weight change in a 5-year prospective analysis of adolescents: Project EAT (Eating Among Teens)," *Pediatrics.* 2008;121:e638-645.

Albertson AM, Thompson D, Franko DL, Kleinman RE, Barton BA, Crockett SJ, "Consumption of breakfast cereal is associated with positive health outcomes: evidence from the National Heart, Lung, and Blood Institute Growth and Health Study," *Nutr Res.* 2008;28:744-752.

De la Hunty A. Gibson S, Ashwell M, "Does regular breakfast cereal consumption help children and adolescents stay slimmer? A systematic review and meta-analysis," *Obes Facts.* 2013;6(1):70-85.

Habit 8: Read the Label

Ollberding NJ1, Wolf RL, Contento I, "Food label use and its relation to dietary intake among US adults," *J Am Diet Assoc.* 2010 Aug;110(8):1233-7.

Borushek A, *The CalorieKing Calorie, Fat & Carbohydrate Counter.* Costa Mesa, California: Family Health Publications, 2014.

Taylor CL, Wilkening VL, "How the nutrition food label was developed, part 1: The Nutrition Facts Panel," *J Am Diet Assoc.* 2008;108:437–442.

Blitstein JL, Evans WD, "Use of nutrition facts panels among adults who make household food purchasing decisions," *J Nutr Educ Behav.* 2006;38:360–364.

Byrd-Bredbenner C, Alfieri L, Kiefer L, "The nutrition label knowledge and usage behaviours of women in the US," *Nutr Bull.* 2000;25:315–322.

Ollberding NJ, Wolf RL, Contento I, "Food label use and its relation to dietary intake among US adults," *J Am Diet Assoc.* 2010;110:1233–1237.

Campos S, Doxey J, Hammond D, "Nutrition labels on pre-packaged foods: a systematic review," *Public Health Nutr.* 2011;14:1496–1506.

Park Y, Subar AF, Hollenbeck A, Schatzkin A. "Dietary fiber intake and mortality in the NIH-AARP diet and health study," *Arch Intern Med.* 2011 Jun 27;171(12): 1061-8.

Cowburn G, Stockley L, "Consumer understanding and use of nutrition labelling: a systematic review," *Public Health Nutr.* 2005;8:21–28.

Pettigrew S, Pescud M, "The salience of food labeling among low-income families with overweight children," *J Nutr Educ Behav.* 2013;45:332–339.

Bryant R, Dundes L, "Portion distortion: a study of college students," *J Consum Aff.* 2005;39:399–408.

Wansink B, Chandon P, "Can 'low-fat' nutrition labels lead to obesity?" *J Marketing Res* 2006; 43: 605–617.

Pelletier AL, Chang WW, Delzell JE, McCall JW, "Patients' understanding and use of snack food package nutrition labels," *J Am Board Fam Pract.* 2004;17:319–323.

Rothman RL, Housam R, Weiss H, Davis D, Gregory R, Gebretsadik T, et al, "Patient understanding of food labels: the role of literacy and numeracy," *Am J Prev Med.* 2006;31:391–398.

Habit 9: Guide to Healthy Restaurant Eating

Nguyen BT, Powell LM, "The impact of restaurant consumption among US adults: effects on energy and nutrient intakes," *Public Health Nutr.* 2014 Nov;17(11):2445-52.

Cohen DA, Bhatia R, "Nutrition standards for away-from-home foods in the USA," *Obes Rev.* 2012 Jul;13(7):618-29.

Powell LM1, Nguyen BT, "Fast-food and full-service restaurant consumption among children and adolescents: effect on energy, beverage, and nutrient intake," *JAMA Pediatr.* 2013 Jan;167(1):14-20.

Guthrie JF, Lin BH, Frazao E, "Role of food prepared away from home in the American diet, 1977-78 versus 1994-96: changes and consequences," *J Nutr Educ Behav.* 2002;34(3):140-150.

Poti JM, Popkin BM, "Trends in energy intake among US children by eating location and food source, 1977-2006," *J Am Diet Assoc.* 2011;111(8):1156-1164.

Vartanian LR, Schwartz MB, Brownell KD, "Effects of soft drink consumption on nutrition and health: a systematic review and meta-analysis," *Am J Public Health.* 2007;97(4):667-675.

Zenk SN, Powell LM, "US secondary schools and food outlets," *Health Place.* 2008;14(2):336-346.

Simon PA, Kwan D, Angelescu A, Shih M, Fielding JE, "Proximity of fast food restaurants to schools: do neighborhood income and type of school matter?" *Prev Med.* 2008;47(3):284-288.

Davis BP, Carpenter CP, "Proximity of fast-food restaurants to schools and adolescent obesity," *Am J Public Health.* 2009;99(3):505-510.

Fleischhacker SE, Evenson KR, Rodriguez DA, Ammerman AS, "A systematic review of fast food access studies," *Obes Rev.* 2011;12(5):e460-e471.

Habit 10: Prepare Your Own Food

Pollan M, *The Omnivore's Dilemma: A Natural History of Four Meals.* New York, New York. Penguin Press, 2006.

Foster GD, Wyatt HR, Hill JO, et al, "Weight and Metabolic Outcomes After 2 Years on a Low-Carbohydrate Versus Low-Fat Diet," *Ann Intern Med.* 2010;153(3):147–155.

Tsai AG, Wadden TA, "Systematic review: an evaluation of major commercial weight loss programs in the United States," *Ann Intern Med.* 2005;142(1):56–66.

Delahanty LM, Conroy MB, Nathan DM, "Psychological predictors of physical activity in the diabetes prevention program," *J Am Diet Assoc.* 2006;106(5):698–705.

Teixeira PJ, Going SB, Houtkooper LB, et al, "Exercise motivation, eating, and body image variables as predictors of weight control," *Med Sci Sports Exerc.* 2006;38(1):179–188.

Teixeira PJ, Palmeira AL, Branco TL, et al, "Who will lose weight? A reexamination of predictors of weight loss in women," *Int J Behav Nutr Phys Act.* 2004;1(1):12.

Kruger J, Galuska DA, Serdula MK, Jones DA, "Attempting to lose weight: specific practices among U.S. adults," *Am J Prev Med.* 2004;26(5):402–406.

Mesas AE, Muñoz-Pareja M, López-García E, Rodríguez-Artalejo F, "Selected eating behaviours and excess body weight: a systematic review," *Obesity Reviews.* 2012;13(2):106–135.

Wyatt HR, Grunwald GK, Mosca CL, et al, "Long-term weight loss and breakfast in subjects in the National Weight Control Registry," *Obes Res.* 2002;10(2):78–82.

Song WO, Chun OK, Obayashi S, Cho S, Chung CE, "Is consumption of breakfast associated with body mass index in US adults?" *J Am Diet Assoc.* 2005;105(9):1373–1382.

Pereira MA, Kartashov AI, Ebbeling CB, et al, "Fast-food habits, weight gain, and insulin resistance (the CARDIA study): 15-year prospective analysis," *Lancet.* 2005;365(9453):36–42.

Imayama I, Alfano CM, Kong A, et al, "Dietary weight loss and exercise interventions effects on quality of life in overweight/obese postmenopausal women: a randomized controlled trial," *Int J Behav Nutr Phys Act.* 2011;8:118.

Mason C, Foster-Schubert KE, Imayama I, et al, "Dietary Weight Loss and Exercise Effects on Insulin Resistance in Postmenopausal Women," *Am J Prev Med.* 2011;41(4):366–375.

Dave JM, An LC, Jeffery RW, Ahluwalia JS, "Relationship of Attitudes Toward Fast Food and Frequency of Fast-food Intake in Adults," *Obesity.* 2009;17(6):1164–1170.

Van der Horst K, Brunner TA, Siegrist M, "Fast food and take-away food consumption are associated with different lifestyle characteristics," *J Hum Nutr Diet.* 2011;24(6):596–602.

Goldstone AP, Prechtl de Hernandez CG, Beaver JD, et al, "Fasting biases brain reward systems towards high-calorie foods," *Eur J Neurosci.* 2009;30(8):1625–1635.

Habit 11: Eat the Clean Calories

Curl CL, Beresford SA, Fenske RA, Fitzpatrick AL, Lu C, Nettleton JA, Kaufman JD, "Estimating Pesticide Exposure from Dietary Intake and Organic Food Choices: The Multi-Ethnic Study of Atherosclerosis (MESA)," *Environ Health Perspect.* 2015 May;123(5):475-83.

Grindler NM, Allsworth JE, Macones GA, Kannan K, Roehl KA, Cooper AR, "Persistent Organic Pollutants and Early Menopause in U.S. Women," *PLoS One.* 2015 Jan 28;10(1):e0116057.

Hornung RW, Reed LD, "Estimation of average concentration in the presence of non-detectable values," *Appl Occup Environ Hyg.* 1990;5:46–51.

Jensen AF, Petersen A, Granby K, "Cumulative risk assessment of the intake of organophosphorus and carbamate pesticides in the Danish diet," *Food Addit Contam.* 2003;20(8):776–785.

Koch D, Lu C, Fisker-Andersen J, Jolley L, Fenske RA, "Temporal association of children's pesticide exposure and agricultural spraying: report of a longitudinal biological monitoring study," *Environ Health Perspect.* 2002;110:829–833.

Kwong TC, "Organophosphate pesticides: biochemistry and clinical toxicology," *Ther Drug Monit.* 2002;24(1):144–149.

Wentz I, Nowosadzka M, *Hashimoto's Thyroiditis: Lifestyle Interventions for Finding and Treating the Root Cause.* Boulder, Colorado: Wentz LLC, 2013.

Zepeda L, Li J, "Characteristics of organic food shoppers," *J Agric Appl Econ.* 2007;39:17–28.

Zhang F, Huang CL, Lin BH, Epperson JE, "Modeling fresh organic produce consumption with scanner data: a generalized double hurdle model approach," *Agribusiness.* 2008;24:510–522.

Habit 12: Weigh Yourself Regularly

Hwang KO, Ning J, Trickey AW, Sciamanna CN, "Website usage and weight loss in a free commercial online weight loss program: retrospective cohort study," *J Med Internet Res.* 2013;15(1):e11.

Pacanowski CR, Levitsky DA, "Frequent Self-Weighing and Visual Feedback for Weight Loss in Overweight Adults," *Journal of Obesity.* 2015;2015:763680.

Gokee-Larose J, Gorin AA, Wing RR., "Behavioral self-regulation for weight loss in young adults: a randomized controlled trial," *International Journal of Behavioral Nutrition and Physical Activity.* 2009;6(1):10.

Steinberg DM, Tate DF, Bennett GG, Ennett S, Samuel-Hodge C, Ward DS, "The efficacy of a daily self-weighing weight loss intervention using smart scales and e-mail," *Obesity.* 2013;21(9):1789–1797.

Butryn ML, Phelan S, Hill JO, Wing RR, "Consistent self-monitoring of weight: a key component of successful weight loss maintenance," *Obesity.* 2007;15(12):3091–3096.

Wing RR, Tate DF, Gorin AA, Raynor HA, Fava JL, "A self-regulation program for maintenance of weight loss," *The New England Journal of Medicine.* 2006;355(15):1563–1571.

Zheng Y, Klem ML, Sereika SM, Danford CA, Ewing LJ, Burke LE, "Self-weighing in weight management: a systematic literature review," *Obesity.* 2015;23(2):256–265.

Flegal KM, Carroll D, Kit BK, Ogden CL, "Prevalence of obesity and trends in the distribution of body mass index among US adults, 1999–2010," *Journal of the American Medical Association.* 2012;307(5):491–497.

Levitsky DA, Garay J, Nausbaum M, Neighbors L, DellaValle DM, "Monitoring weight daily blocks the freshman weight gain: a model for combating the epidemic of obesity," *International Journal of Obesity.* 2006;30(6):1003–1010.

Levitsky DA, "The non-regulation of food intake in humans: hope for reversing the epidemic of obesity," *Physiology and Behavior.* 2005;86(5):623–632.

Elfhag K, Rossner S, "Initial weight loss is the best predictor for success in obesity treatment and sociodemographic liabilities increase risk for drop-out," *Patient Education and Counseling.* 2010;79(3):361–366.

Habit 13: Automate Eating

Khaylis A, Yiaslas T, Bergstrom J, Gore-Felton C, "A Review of Efficacious Technology-Based Weight-Loss Interventions: Five Key Components," *Telemedicine Journal and e-Health.* 2010;16(9):931–938.

Berge JM, Wall M, Hsueh TF, Fulkerson JA, Larson N, Neumark-Sztainer D, "The Protective Role of Family Meals for Youth Obesity: 10-Year Longitudinal Associations," *J Pediatr.* 2015 Feb;166(2):296-301.

Flegal KMCM, Ogden CL, "Curtin LR. Prevalence and trends in obesity among US adults, 1999–2008," *JAMA.* 2010;303:235–241.

Eckel RH, Grundy SM, Zimmet PZ, "The metabolic syndrome," *Lancet.* 2005;365:1415–1428.

Greenberg I, Perna F, Kaplan M, Sullivan MA, "Behavioral and psychological factors in assessment and treatment of obesity surgery patients," *Obes Res.* 2005;13:244–249.

Wadden TA, McGuckin B, Wilson C, "Lifestyle modification for the management of obesity," *Gastroenterology.* 2007;132:2226–2238.

Heshka S, Anderson JW, Atkinson RL, et al, "Weight loss with self-help compared with a structured commercial program: a randomized trial," *JAMA.* 2003;289:1792–1798.

Neve M, Morgan PJ, Jones PR, Collins CE, "Effectiveness of web-based interventions in achieving weight-loss and weight-loss maintenance in overweight and obese adults: a systematic review with meta-analysis," *Obes Res.* 2010;11:306–321.

Norman GJ, Zabinski MF, Adams MA, Rosenberg DE, Yaroch AL, Atienza AA, "A review of eHealth interventions for physical activity and dietary behavior change," *Am J Prev Med.* 2007;33:336–345.

Tate DF, Jackvony EH, Wing RR, "Effects of Internet behavioral counseling on weight loss in adults at risk for type 2 diabetes: a randomized trial," *JAMA.* 2003;289:1833–1836.

Bennett GG, Herring SJ, Puleo E, Stein EK, Emmons KM, Gillman MW, "Web-based weight loss in primary care: A randomized controlled trial," *Obesity.* 2010;18:308–313.

Krukowski RA, Harvey-Berino J, Ashikaga T, Thomas CS, Micco N, "Internet-based weight control: The relationship between web features and weight loss," *Telemed J E Health.* 2008;14:775–782.

Polzien KM, Jakicic JM, Tate DF, Otto AD, "The efficacy of a technology-based system in a short-term behavioral weight loss intervention," *Obesity.* 2007;15:825–830.

Micco N, Gold B, Buzzell P, Leonard H, Pintauro S, Harvey-Berino J, "Minimal in-person support as an adjunct to Internet obesity treatment," *Ann Behav Med.* 2007;33:49–56.

Wing RR, Tate DF, Gorin AA, Raynor HA, Fava JL, "A self-regulation program for maintenance of weight loss," *N Engl J Med.* 2006;255:1563–1571.

Rothert, Strecher VJ, Doyle LA, et al, "Web-based weight management programs in an integrated health setting: A randomized, controlled trial," *Obesity.* 2006;14:266–272.

Svetkey LP, Stevens VJ, Brantley PJ, et al, "Comparison of strategies for sustaining weight loss: The weight loss maintenance randomized controlled trial," *JAMA.* 2008;299:1139–1148.

Harvey-Berino J, Pintauro S, Buzzell P, Casey Gold B, "Effect of Internet support on the long-term maintenance of weight loss," *Obes Res.* 2004;12:320–329.

Cussler EC, Teixeira PJ, Going SB, et al, "Maintenance of weight loss in overweight middle-aged women through the Internet," *Obesity.* 2008;16:1052–1060.

Habit 14: Slow Down

Lee S, Ko BJ, Gong Y, Han K, Lee A, Han BD, Yoon YJ, Park S, Kim JH, Mantzoros CS, "Self-reported eating speed in relation to non-alcoholic fatty liver disease in adults," *Eur J Nutr.* 2015 Feb 4.1-7.

Almiron-Roig E, Tsiountsioura M, Lewis HB, Wu J, Solis-Trapala I, Jebb SA, "Large portion sizes increase bite size and eating rate in overweight women," *Physiol Behav.* 2015 Feb;139:297-302.

Shah M, Copeland J, Dart L, Adams-Huet B, James A, Rhea D, "Slower eating speed lowers energy intake in normal-weight but not overweight/obese subjects," *J Acad Nutr Diet.* 2014 Mar;114(3):393-402.

Lee KS, Kim DH, Jang JS, Nam GE, Shin YN, Bok AR, et al, "Eating rate is associated with cardiometabolic risk factors in Korean adults," *Nutr Metab Cardiovasc Dis.* 2013;23:635–641.

Andrade AM, Greene GW, Melanson KJ, "Eating slowly led to decreases in energy intake within meals in healthy women," *J Am Diet Assoc.* 2008 Jul;108(7):1186-91.

Sakurai M, Nakamura K, Miura K, Takamura T, Yoshita K, Nagasawa SY et al, "Self-reported speed of eating and 7-year risk of type 2 diabetes mellitus in middle-aged Japanese men," *Metabolism.* 2006;61:1566–1571.

Michalakis K, Mintziori G, Kaprara A, Tarlatzis BC, Goulis DG, "The complex interaction between obesity, metabolic syndrome and reproductive axis: a narrative review," *Metabolism.* 2013;62:457–478.

Tsatsoulis A, Mantzaris MD, Bellou S, Andrikoula M, "Insulin resistance: an adaptive mechanism becomes maladaptive in the current environment—an evolutionary perspective," *Metabolism.* 2013;62:622–633.

Tanihara S, Imatoh T, Miyazaki M, Babazono A, Momose Y, Baba M, et al, "Retrospective longitudinal study on the relationship between 8-year weight change and current eating speed," *Appetite.* 2011;57:179–183.

Viskaal-van Dongen M, Kok FJ, de Graaf C, "Eating rate of commonly consumed foods promotes food and energy intake," *Appetite.* 2011;56:25–31.

Karl JP, Young AJ, Rood JC, Montain SJ, "Independent and combined effects of eating rate and energy density on energy intake, appetite, and gut hormones," *Obesity.* 2013;21:E244–E252.

Habit 15: Avoid Excessive Alcohol

Bagnardi V1, Blangiardo M, La Vecchia C, Corrao G, "Alcohol consumption and the risk of cancer: a meta-analysis," *Alcohol Res Health.* 2001;25(4):263-70.

Pelucchi C, Tramacere I, Boffetta P, Negri E, La Vecchia C, "Alcohol consumption and cancer risk," *Nutr Cancer.* 2011;63(7):983-90.

Vogel RA, "Alcohol, heart disease, and mortality: a review," *Rev Cardiovasc Med.* 2002 Winter;3(1):7-13.

Secretan B, Straif K, Baan R, Grosse Y, Ghissassi F, "A review of human carcinogens—Part E: tobacco, areca nut, alcohol, coal smoke, and salted fish," *Lancet Oncol.* 2009;10:1033–1034.

Allen, N E, Beral, V, Casabonne, D, Kan, S W Reeves, G K, "Moderate alcohol intake and cancer incidence in women," *J Natl Cancer Inst.* 2009;101:296–305.

Enzinger PC, Mayer, RJ, "Esophageal cancer," *N Engl J Med.* 2003;349:2241–2252.

Jepsen P, Johnsen SP, Gillman MW, Sorensen HT, "Interpretation of observational studies," *Heart.* 2004 Aug; 90(8):956–960.

Herrington DM, "Hormone replacement therapy and heart disease: replacing dogma with data," *Circulation.* 2003 Jan 7;107(1):2-4.

Liang H, Wang J, Xiao H, Wang D, Wei W, "Estimation of cancer incidence and mortality attributable to alcohol drinking in China," *BMC Public Health.* 2010;10:730.

Bagnardi V, Blangiardo M, La Vecchia C, Corrao G, "A meta-analysis of alcohol drinking and cancer risk," *Br J Cancer.* 2001;85:1700–1705.

Islami F, Tramacere I, Rota M, Bagnardi V, Fedirko V, "Alcohol drinking and laryngeal cancer: overall and dose-risk relation—a systematic review and meta-analysis," *Oral Oncol.* 2010;46:802–810.

Tramacere I, Negri E, Bagnardi V, Garavello W, Rota M, "A meta-analysis of alcohol drinking and oral and pharyngeal cancers. Part 1: overall results and dose-risk relation," *Oral Oncol.* 2010;46:497–503.

Turati F, Garavello W, Tramacere I, et al, "A meta-analysis of alcohol drinking and oral and pharyngeal cancers. Part 2: results by subsites," *Oral Oncol.* 2010;46:720–726.

Bagnardi V, Zambon A, Quatto P, Corrao G, "Flexible meta-regression functions for modeling aggregate dose-response data, with an application to alcohol and mortality," *Am J Epidemiol.* 2004;159:1077–1086.

Pelucchi C, Gallus S, Garavello W, Bosetti C, La Vecchia C, "Alcohol and tobacco use, and cancer risk for upper aerodigestive tract and liver," *Eur J Cancer Prev.* 2008;17:340–344.

Boffetta P, Hashibe M, La Vecchia C, Zatonski W, Rehm J, "The burden of cancer attributable to alcohol drinking," *Int J Cancer.* 2006;119:884–887.

Exercise

Habit 16: Practice Regular Physical Activity

Conroy MB, Yang K, Elci OU, et al, "Physical activity self-monitoring and weight loss: 6-month results of the SMART trial," *Med Sci Sports Exerc.* 2011;43(8):1568–1574.

Ratey J, Hagerman E, *Spark: The Revolutionary New Science of Exercise and the Brain.* New York, New York: Little Brown & Company, 2013.

Sugden JA, Sniehotta FF, Donnan PT, Boyle P, Johnston DW, McMurdo MET, "The feasibility of using pedometers and brief advice to increase activity in sedentary older women—a pilot study," *BMC Health Serv Res.* 2008;8:169.

Carels RA, Darby LA, Rydin S, Douglass OM, Cacciapaglia HM, O'Brien WH, "The relationship between self-monitoring, outcome expectancies, difficulties with eating and exercise, and physical activity and weight loss treatment outcomes," *Ann Behav Med.* 2005;30(3):182–190.

Lee LL, Kuo YC, Fanaw D, Perng SJ, Juang IF, "The effect of an intervention combining self-efficacy theory and pedometers on promoting physical activity among adolescents," *J Clin Nurs.* 2012 Apr;21(7-8):914-22.

Tudor-Locke C, Lutes L, "Why do pedometers work?" *Sports Med.* 2009;39(12):981–993.

Ainsworth B, Haskell WL, White MC, et al, "Compendium of physical activities: an update of activity codes and MET intensities," *Med Sci Sports Exerc.* 2000;32(Suppl):S498–S504.

Baker RC, Kirschenbaum DS, "Self-monitoring may be necessary for successful weight control," *Behavior Therapy.* 1993;24:377–394.

Burke LE, Warziski M, Styn MA, Music E, Hudson AG, Sereika SM, "A randomized clinical trial of a standard versus vegetarian diet for weight loss: The impact of treatment preference," *International Journal of Obesity.* 2008;32:166–176.

Burke LE, Swigart V, Warziski Turk M, Derro N, Ewing LJ, "Experiences of self-monitoring: successes and struggles during treatment for weight loss," *Qual Health Res.* 2009 Jun;19(6):815–28.

Tudor-Locke C, Johnson WD, Katzmarzyk PT, "Accelerometer-determined steps per day in US adults," *Med Sci Sports Exerc.* 2009;41:1384–1391.

Tudor-Locke C, "Steps to better cardiovascular health: how many steps does it take to achieve good health and how confident are we in this number?" *Curr Cardiovasc Risk Rep.* 2010;4:271–276.

Tudor-Locke C, Bassett DR, "How many steps/day are enough? Preliminary pedometer indices for public health," *Sports Med.* 2004;34:1–8.

Tudor-Locke C, Hatano Y, Pangrazi RP, Kang M, "Revisiting "How many steps are enough?"." *Med Sci Sports Exerc.* 2008;40:S537–543.

Tudor-Locke C, Craig CL, Beets MW, Belton S, Cardon GM, Duncan S, Hatano Y, Lubans DR, Olds TS, Raustorp A. et al, "How many steps/day are enough? For children and adolescents," *Int J Behav Nutr Phys Act.* 2011;8:78.

Tudor-Locke C, Craig CL, Aoyagi Y, Bell RC, Croteau KA, De Bourdeaudhuij I, Ewald B, Gardner AW, Hatano Y, Lutes LD, et al, "How many steps/day are enough? For older adults and special populations," *Int J Behav Nutr Phys Act.* 2011;8(1):80.

McCormack G, Giles-Corti B, Milligan R, "Demographic and individual correlates of achieving 10,000 steps/day: use of pedometers in a population-based study," *Health Promot J Austr.* 2006;17:43–47.

Tudor-Locke C, Bassett DR, Shipe MF, McClain JJ, "Pedometry methods for assessing free-living adults," *J Phys Act Health.* 2011;8:445–453.

Krumm EM, Dessieux OL, Andrews P, Thompson DL, "The relationship between daily steps and body composition in postmenopausal women," *J Womens Health.* 2006;15:202–210.

Schmidt MD, Cleland VJ, Shaw K, Dwyer T, Venn AJ, "Cardiometabolic risk in younger and older adults across an index of ambulatory activity," *Am J Prev Med.* 2009;37:278–284.

Habit 17: The Importance of Aerobic Exercise

Jakicic JM, Marcus BH, Lang W, Janney C, "Effect of exercise on 24-month weight loss maintenance in overweight women," *Arch. Intern. Med.* 2008;168(14):1550–9.

Macneil I, *The Sports Medicine Council of British Columbia. The Beginning Runner's Handbook:*

The Proven 13-Week RunWalk Program. Vancouver BC, Canada: Greystone Books, 2012.

Bingham J. *The Courage To Start: A Guide To Running for Your Life.* New York, New York: Fireside, 1999.

Pang MY1, Charlesworth SA, Lau RW, Chung RC, "Using aerobic exercise to improve health outcomes and quality of life in stroke: evidence-based exercise prescription recommendations," *Cerebrovasc Dis.* 2013;35(1):7-22.

Lee VL, Foody JM, "Women and heart disease," *Cardiol Clin.* 2001;29:35–45.

Zhang C, Rexrode KM, vanDam RM, Li TY, Hu FB, "Abdominal obesity and risk of all cause cardiovascular and cancer mortality," *Circulation.* 2008;117:1658–1667.

deGonzalez A, Hartge P, Cerhan JR, Flint AJ, Hannan L, MacInnis RJ, et al, "Body-mass index and mortality among 1.46 million white adults," *New Engl J Med.* 2010;363:2211–2219.

Vaccarino V, McClure C, Johnson D, Sheps DS, Bittner V, Rutledge T, et al, "Depression: the metabolic syndrome and cardiovascular risk," *Psychosomatic Med.* 2008;70:40–48.

Berger JS, Jordan CO, Lloyd-Jones D, Blumenthal RS, "Screening for cardiovascular risk in asymptomatic patients," *J Am Coll Cardiol.* 2010;531:169–1177.

Demark-Wahnefried W, Jones LW, "Promoting a healthy lifestyle among cancer survivors," *Hematol Oncol Clin N Am.* 2008;22:319–42.

Morey MC, Snyder DC, Sloane R, Cohen HJ, Peterson B, Hartman TJ, "Effects of home-based diet and exercise on functional outcomes among older, overweight long-term cancer survivors: RENEW: A randomized controlled trial," *JAMA.* 2009;301:1883–91.

Jakicic JM, Marcus BH, Gallagher KI, Napolitano M, Lang W, "Effect of exercise duration and intensity on weight loss in overweight, sedentary women. A randomized trial," *JAMA.* 2003;290:1323–1330.

Saris WHM, Blair SN, van Baak MA, et al, "How much physical activity is enough to prevent unhealthy weight gain? Outcome of the IASO 1st Stock Conference and consensus statement," *Obesity Reviews.* 2003;4:101–114.

Wing RR, Tate DF, Gorin AA, Raynor HA, Fava JL, "A self-regulation program for maintenance of weight loss," *N Engl J Med.* 2006;355:1563–1571.

Habit 18: Weight Training

Westcott WL, "Resistance training is medicine: effects of strength training on health," *Curr Sports Med Rep.* 2012 Jul-Aug;11(4):209-16.

Hurley BF1, Hanson ED, Sheaff AK, "Strength training as a countermeasure to aging muscle and chronic disease, *Sports Med.* 2011 Apr 1;41(4):289-306.

Phillips, B, *Body for Life: 12 Weeks to Mental and Physical Strength.* New York, New York: Harper Collins, 1999.

Peeke P, *Body for Life for Women: A Woman's Plan for Physical and Mental Transformation.* Emmaus, PA: Rodale, 2005.

Blair SN, Kohl HW, Barlow CE, et al, "Changes in physical fitness and all-cause mortality: a prospective study of healthy and unhealthy men," *JAMA.* 1995;273:1093–8.

Wolfe RR, "The underappreciated role of muscle in health and disease," *Am J Clin Nutr.* 2006;84:475–82.

Suetta C, Magnusson SP, Beyer N, et al, "Effect of strength training on muscle function in elderly hospitalized patients," *Scand J Med Sci Sports.* 2007;17:464–72.

Tanasescu M, Leitzmann MF, Rimm EB, et al, "Exercise type and intensity in relation to coronary heart disease in men," *JAMA.* 2002;288(16):1994–2000.

Braith RW, Stewart KJ, "Resistance exercise training: its role in the prevention of cardiovascular disease," *Circulation.* 2006;113:2642–50.

Evans WJ, "Skeletal muscle loss: cachexia, sarcopenia, and inactivity," *Am J Clin Nutr.* 2010;91:1123–7S.

Melov S, Tarnopolsky MA, Beckman K, et al, "Resistance exercise reverses aging in human skeletal muscle," *PLoS One.* 2007;2:(5):E465.

DiPenta JM, Green-Johnson JM, Murphy RJ, "Type 2 diabetes mellitus, resistance training, and innate immunity: is there a common link?" *Appl Physiol Nutr Metab.* 2007;32:1025–35.

Murphy JL, Blakely EL, Schaefer AM, et al, "Resistance training in patients with single, large-scale deletions of mitochondrial DNA," *Brain.* 2008;131:2832–40.

Johnston AP, De LM, Parise G, "Resistance training, sarcopenia, and the mitochondrial theory of aging," *Appl Physiol Nutr Metab.* 2008;33:191–9.

Petersen KF, Befroy D, Dufour S, et al, "Mitochondrial dysfunction in the elderly: possible role in insulin resistance," *Science* 2003;300:1140–2.

Alberti KG, Zimmet P, Shaw J, "Metabolic syndrome: a new world-wide definition. A Consensus Statement from The International Diabetes Federation," *Diabet Med.* 2006;23:469–80.

Reaven G, "The metabolic syndrome or the insulin resistance syndrome? Different names, different concepts, and different goals," *Endocrinol Metab Clin North Am.* 2004;33:283–303.

Close GL, Kayani A, Vasilaki A, et al, "Skeletal muscle damage with exercise and aging," *Sports Med* 2005;35:413–27.

Tresierras MA, Balady GJ, "Resistance training in the treatment of diabetes and obesity: mechanisms and outcomes," *J Cardiopulm Rehabil Prev.* 2009;29:67–75.

Smith Jr SC, "Multiple risk factors for cardiovascular disease and diabetes mellitus," *Am J Med* 2007;120:S3–11.

Li C, Ford ES, McGuire LC, et al, "Increasing trends in waist circumference and abdominal obesity among U.S. adults," *Obesity.* 2007;15:216–24.

Pighon A, Paquette A, Barsalani R, et al, "Substituting food restriction by resistance training prevents liver and body fat regain in ovariectomized rats," *Climacteric.* 2009;12:153–64.

Kotronen A, Yki-Jarvinen H, "Fatty liver: a novel component of the metabolic syndrome," *Arterioscler Thromb Vasc Biol.* 2008;28:27–38.

Buchman AS, Schneider JA, Leurgans S, et al, "Physical frailty in older persons is associated with Alzheimer disease pathology," *Neurology.* 2008;71:499–504.

Lachman ME, Neupert SD, Bertrand R, et al, "The effects of strength training on memory in older adults," *J Aging Phys Act.* 2006;14:59–73.

Cassilhas RC, Viana VA, Grassmann V, et al, "The impact of resistance exercise on the cognitive function of the elderly," *Med Sci Sports Exerc.* 2007;39:1401–7.

Liu-Ambrose T, Donaldson MG, "Exercise and cognition in older adults: is there a role for resistance training programmes?" *Br J Sports Med.* 2009;43:25–7.

Sigal RJ, Kenny GP, Boule NG, et al, "Effects of aerobic training, resistance training, or both on glycemic control in type 2 diabetes: a randomized trial," *Ann Intern Med.* 2007;147:357–69.

Habit 19: Stretch

Page P, "Current concepts in muscle stretching for exercise and rehabilitation," *Int J Sports Phys Ther.* 2012 Feb;7(1):109-19.

McHugh MP, Cosgrave CH, "To stretch or not to stretch: the role of stretching in injury prevention and performance," *Scandinavian journal of medicine & science in sports.* 2010 Apr;20(2):169–181.

Small K, Mc NL, Matthews M, "A systematic review into the efficacy of static stretching as part of a warm-up for the prevention of exercise-related injury," *Res Sports Med.* 2008 Jul;16(3):213–231.

Thacker SB, Gilchrist J, Stroup DF, Kimsey CD., Jr, "The impact of stretching on sports injury risk: a systematic review of the literature," *Med Sci Sports Exerc.* 2004 Mar;36(3):371–378.

Ylinen J, Kankainen T, Kautiainen H, Rezasoltani A, Kuukkanen T, Hakkinen A, "Effect of stretching on hamstring muscle compliance," *J Rehabil Med.* 2009 Jan;41(1):80–84.

McHugh MP, Nesse M, "Effect of stretching on strength loss and pain after eccentric exercise," *Med Sci Sports Exerc.* 2008 Mar;40(3):566–573.

Behm DG, Kibele A, "Effects of differing intensities of static stretching on jump performance," *Eur J Appl Physiol.* 2007 Nov;101(5):587–594.

Ce E, Margonato V, Casasco M, Veicsteinas A, "Effects of stretching on maximal anaerobic power: the roles of active and passive warm-ups," *J Strength Cond Res.* 2008 May;22(3):794–800.

Sayers AL, Farley RS, Fuller DK, Jubenville CB, Caputo JL, "The effect of static stretching on phases of sprint performance in elite soccer players," *J Strength Cond Res.* 2008 Sep;22(5):1416–1421.

Behm D, Button DC, Butt JC, "Factors affecting force loss with prolonged stretching," *Can J Appl Physiol.* 2001;26(3):262–272.

Torres EM, Kraemer WJ, Vingren JL, et al, "Effects of stretching on upper-body muscular performance," *J Strength Cond Res.* 2008 Jul;22(4):1279–1285.

Yamaguchi T, Ishii K, "Effects of static stretching for 30 seconds and dynamic stretching on leg extension power," *J Strength Cond Res.* 2005 Aug;19(3):677–683.

Pearce AJ, Kidgell DJ, Zois J, Carlson JS, "Effects of secondary warm up following stretching," *Eur J Appl Physiol.* 2009 Jan;105(2):175–183.

Habit 20: Meditate

Astin JA, Shapiro SL, Eisenberg DM, Forys KL, "Mind-body medicine: state of the science, implications for practice," *J Am Board Fam Pract.* 2003;16(2):131-47.

Benson H, *The Relaxation Response.* New York, New York: Harper Collins, 1975.

Benson H, Stark M, *Timeless Healing: The Power and Biology of Belief.* New York, New York: Simon & Schuster, 1996.

Dusek JA, Benson H, "Mind-Body Medicine. A Model of the Comparative Clinical Impact of the Acute Stress and Relaxation Responses," *Minn Med.* 2009 May;92(5):47–50.

Easwaran E, *Meditation: A Simple Eight-Point Program for Translating Spiritual Ideals into Daily Life*. Tomales, California: Nilgiri Press, 1991.

LeShan L, *How To Meditate: A Guide To Self-Discovery*. Boston, Massachusetts: Little Brown & Company, 1974.

Schneider RH, Grim CE, Rainforth MV, Kotchen T, Nidich SI, Gaylord-King C, Salerno JW, Kotchen JM, Alexander CN, "Meditation programs for psychological stress and well-being: a systematic review and meta-analysis," *JAMA*. 2014 Mar;174(3):357-68.

Rapgay L, Bystrisky A, "Classical mindfulness: an introduction to its theory and practice for clinical application," *Ann N.Y. Acad Sci*. 2009 Aug;1172:148-162.

Chiesa A, Malinowski P, "Mindfulness-based approaches: are they all the same?" *J Clin Psychol*. 2011;67(4):404-424.

Sedlmeier P, Eberth J, Schwarz M, et al, "The psychological effects of meditation: a meta-analysis," *Psychol Bull*. 2012;138(6):1139-1171.

Bohlmeijer E, Prenger R, Taal E, Cuijpers P, "The effects of mindfulness-based stress reduction therapy on mental health of adults with a chronic medical disease: a meta-analysis," *J Psychosom Res*. 2010;68(6):539-544.

Chambers R, Gullone E, Allen NB, "Mindful emotion regulation: an integrative review," *Clin Psychol Rev*. 2009;29(6):560-572.

Chiesa A, Serretti A, "Mindfulness based cognitive therapy for psychiatric disorders: a systematic review and meta-analysis," *Psychiatry Res*. 2011;187(3):441-453.

Hofmann SG, Sawyer AT, Witt AA, Oh D, "The effect of mindfulness-based therapy on anxiety and depression: a meta-analytic review," *J Consult Clin Psychol*. 2010;78(2):169-183.

Krisanaprakornkit T, Ngamjarus C, Witoonchart C, Piyavhatkul N, "Meditation therapies for attention-deficit/hyperactivity disorder (ADHD)," *Cochrane Database Syst Rev*. 2010;(6):CD006507.

Ledesma D, Kumano H, "Mindfulness-based stress reduction and cancer: a meta-analysis," *Psychooncology*. 2009;18(6):571-579.

Wanden-Berghe RG, Sanz-Valero J, Wanden-Berghe C, "The application of mindfulness to eating disorders treatment: a systematic review," *Eat Disord*. 2011;19(1):34-48.

Zgierska A, Rabago D, Chawla N, Kushner K, Koehler R, Marlatt A, "Mindfulness meditation for substance use disorders: a systematic review," *Subst Abus*. 2009;30(4):266-294.

Personal

Habit 21: Plan Your Calendar Weekly

Covey, SR, Merrill, RA, Merrill, RR, *First Things First: To Live, To Learn, to Leave a Legacy*. New York, New York: Simon & Schuster, 1994.

Allen D, *Getting Things Done: The Art of Stress-Free Productivity*. New York, New York: Penguin Books, 2001.

Habit 22: Practice Good Dental Hygiene

Montebugnoli L1, Servidio D, Miaton RA, Prati C, Tricoci P, Melloni C, Poor oral health is associated with coronary heart disease and elevated systemic inflammatory and haemostatic factors," *J Clin Periodontol.* 2004 Jan;31(1):25-9.

Kaisare S1, Rao J, Dubashi, "Periodontal disease as a risk factor for acute myocardial infarction. A case-control study in Goans highlighting a review of the literature," *Br Dent J.* 2007 Aug 11;203(3):E5; discussion 144-5.

Lynch H, Milgrom P, "Xylitol and dental caries: an overview for clinicians," *J Calif Dent Assoc.* 2003 Mar;31(3):205-9.

Holmstrup P, Poulsen AH, Andersen L, Skuldbol T, Fiehn NE, "Oral infections and systemic diseases," *Dent Clin North Am.* 2003;47:575–98.

Hujoel PP, Drangsholt M, Spiekerman C, Derouen TA, "Examining the link between coronary heart disease and the elimination of chronic dental infections," *J Am Dent Assoc.* 2001;132:883–9.

Howell TH, Ridker PM, Ajani UA, Hennekens CH, Christen WG, "Periodontal disease and risk of subsequent cardiovascular disease in U.S. male physicians," *J Am Coll Cardiol.* 2001;37:445–50.

Tuominen R, Reunanen A, Paunio M, Paunio I, Aromaa A, "Oral health indicators poorly predict coronary heart disease deaths," *J Dent Res.* 2003;82:713–8.

Stein JM, Kuch B, Conrads G, Fickl S, Chrobot J, Schulz S, et al, "Clinical periodontal and microbiologic parameters in patients with acute myocardial infarction," *J Periodontol.* 2009;80:1581–9.

Armitage GC, "Periodontal infections and cardiovascular disease—How strong is the association?" *Oral Dis.* 2000;6:335–50.

Janket SJ, Baird AE, Chuang SK, Jones JA, "Meta-analysis of periodontal disease and risk of coronary heart disease and stroke," *Oral Surg Oral Med Oral Pathol Oral Radiol Endod.* 2003;95:559–69.

Rutger PG, Ohlsson O, Pettersson T, Renvert S, "Chronic periodontitis, a significant relationship with acute myocardial infarction," *Eur Heart J.* 2003;24:2108–15.

Cueto A, Mesa F, Bravo M, Ocaña-Riola R, "Periodontitis as risk factor for acute myocardial infarction. A case control study of Spanish adults," *J Periodontal Res.* 2005;40:36–42.

Rai B, Kaur J, Jain RK, Anand SC, "Periodontal disease and coronary heart disease," JK Sci. 2009;11:194–5.

Vijayalakshmi R, Anitha S, Emmadi P, Ambalavanan N, Ramarishnan T, Saravankumar R, "Association between periodontal disease and acute myocardial infarction," *J Ind Assoc Public Health Dent.* 2007;10:101–6.

Habit 23: Practice Safe Driving Habits

Llerena LE, Aronow KV, Macleod J, Bard M, Salzman S, Greene W, Haider A, Schupper A, "An evidence-based review: distracted driver," *J Trauma Acute Care Surg.* 2015 Jan;78(1):147-52.

Irwin C, Monement S, Desbrow B, "The influence of drinking, texting, and eating on simulated driving performance," *Traffic Inj Prev.* 2015;16(2):116-23.

Fitch GA, Soccolich SA, Guo F, McClaffert, Y J, Fang Y, Olson RL, Perez MA, Hanowski RJ, Hankey JM, Dingus TA, *The impact of hand-held and hands-free cell phone use on driving performance and safety-critical event risk.* 2013. Washington, DC: National Highway Traffic Safety Administration.

McKeever JD, Schultheis MT, Padmanaban V, Blasco A, "Driver performance while texting: even a little is too much," *Traffic Inj Prev.* 2013;14(2):132-7.

McEvoy SP, Stevenson MR, McCartt AT, et al, "Role of mobile phones in motor vehicle crashes resulting in hospital attendance: a case-crossover study," *BMJ.* 2005;331:428.

Young KL, Salmon PM, Cornelissen M, "Missing links? The effects of distraction on driver situation awareness," *Safety Science.* 2013;56:36–43.

Neyens DM, Boyle LN, "The effect of distractions on the crash types of teenage drivers," *Accident Analysis and Prevention.* 2007;39(1):206–212.

Recarte MA, Nunes LM, "Mental Workload While Driving: Effects on Visual Search, Discrimination, and Decision Making," *Journal of Experimental Psychology.* 2003;9(2):119–137.

Lee JD, Caven B, Haake S, Brown TL, "Speech-based interaction with in-vehicle computers: The effect of speech-based e-mail on drivers' attention to the roadway," *Human Factors.* 2001;43(4):631–640.

Liang Y, Lee JD, Yekhshatyan L, "How dangerous is looking away from the road? Algorithms predict crash risk from glance patterns in naturalistic driving," *Human Factors.* 2012;54(6):1104–1116.

Lee SE, Simons-Morton BG, Klauer SE, Ouimet MC, Dingus TA, "Naturalistic assessment of novice teenage crash experience," *Accident Analysis and Prevention.* 2011;43(4):1472–1479.

Guo F, Klauer SG, Hankey JM, Dingus TA, "Near crashes as crash surrogate for naturalistic driving studies," *Journal of the Transportation Research Board.* 2010;(2147):66–74.

Horrey WJ, Lesch MF, Garabet A, "Assessing the awareness of performance decrements in distracted drivers," *Accident Analysis and Prevention.* 2008;40(2):675–682.

Chan E, Pradhan AK, Knodler MA, Pollatsek A, Fisher DL, *Empirical Evaluation on a Driving Simulator of the Effect of Distractions Inside and Outside the Vehicle on Drivers' Eye Behaviors.* Washington, D.C.: National Research Council, 2008.

Governors Highway Safety Association http://www.ghsa.org

CDC Driver Safety Website: http://www.cdc.gov/motorvehiclesafety/

Habit 24: Anticipation

Vilhauer J, *Think Forward to Thrive: How to Use the Mind's Power of Anticipation to Transcend Your Past and Transform Your Life.* Novato, California: New World Library, 2014.

Habit 25: Do Not Smoke

Carter BD, Abnet CC, Feskanich D, Freedman ND, Hartge P, Lewis CE, Ockene JK, Prentice RL, Speizer FE, Thun MJ, Jacobs EJ, "Smoking and mortality--beyond established causes," *N Engl J Med.* 2015 Feb 12;372(7):631-40.

The health consequences of smoking: 50 years of progress: a report of the Surgeon General. Department of Health and Human Services, Centers for Disease Control and Prevention, National Center for Chronic Disease Prevention and Health Promotion, Office on Smoking and Health, 2014 www.surgeongeneral.gov/library/reports/50-years-of-progress/#fullreport

Pirie K, Peto R, Reeves GK, Green J, Beral V, "The 21st century hazards of smoking and benefits of stopping: a prospective study of one million women in the UK," *Lancet.* 2013;381:133-141.

Thun MJ, Carter BD, Feskanich D, et al, "50-Year trends in smoking-related mortality in the United States," *N Engl J Med.* 2013;368:351-364.

Calle EE, Rodriguez C, Jacobs EJ, et al, "The American Cancer Society Cancer Prevention Study II nutrition cohort: rationale, study design, and baseline characteristics," *Cancer.* 2002;94:2490-2501.

Unal B, Bilgili MY, Yilmaz S, Caglayan O, Kara S, "Smoking prevents the expected postprandial increase in intestinal blood flow: a Doppler sonographic study," *J Ultrasound Med.* 2004;23:647-653.

Arcavi L, Benowitz NL, "Cigarette smoking and infection," *Arch Intern Med.* 2004;164:2206-2216.

Bagaitkar J, Demuth DR, Scott DA, "Tobacco use increases susceptibility to bacterial infection," *Tob Induc Dis.* 2008;4:12.

Zhang L, Ren JW, Wong CC, et al, "Effects of cigarette smoke and its active components on ulcer formation and healing in the gastrointestinal mucosam," *Curr Med Chem.* 2012;19:63-69.

Sadr-Azodi O, Andrén-Sandberg A, Orsini N, Wolk A, "Cigarette smoking, smoking cessation and acute pancreatitis: a prospective population-based study," *Gut.* 2012;61:262-267.

Secretan B, Straif K, Baan R, et al, "A review of human carcinogens," *Lancet Oncol.* 2009;10:1033-1034.

Gaudet MM, Gapstur SM, Sun J, Diver WR, Hannan LM, Thun MJ, "Active smoking and breast cancer risk: original cohort data and meta-analysis," *J Natl Cancer Inst.* 2013;105:515-525.

Bryan L, Westmaas L, Alcaraz K, Jemal A, "Cigarette smoking and cancer screening underutilization by state: BRFSS 2010," *Nicotine Tob Res.* 2014;16:1183-1189.

Huncharek M, Haddock KS, Reid R, Kupelnick B, "Smoking as a risk factor for prostate cancer: a meta-analysis of 24 prospective cohort studies," *Am J Public Health.* 2010;100:693-701.

Habit 26: Sleep Well

Jacobs, GD, *Say Good Night To Insomnia.* New York, New York: Henry Holt & Company, 1998.

Gelber RP, Redline S, Ross GW, Petrovitch H, Sonnen JA, Zarow C, Uyehara-Lock JH, Masaki KH, Launer LJ, White LR, "Associations of brain lesions at autopsy with polysomnography features before death," *Neurology.* 2015 Jan;84(3): 296-303.

Cappuccio FP, D'Elia L, Strazzullo P, Miller MA, "Quantity and quality of sleep and incidence of type 2 diabetes: a systematic review and meta-analysis," *Diabetes Care.* 2010 Feb;33(2):414-20.

Weissbluth M, *Healthy Sleep Habits, Happy Child: A Step-By-Step Program For A Good Night's Sleep.* New York, New York. Ballantine Publishing Group, 1999.

Mullington JM, Haack M, Toth M, Serrador JM, Meier-Ewert HK, "Cardiovascular, inflammatory, and metabolic consequences of sleep deprivation," *Prog Cardiovasc Dis.* 2009 Jan-Feb;51(4):294-302.

Cappuccio FP, D'Elia L, Strazzullo P, Miller MA, "Sleep duration and all-cause mortality: a systematic review and meta-analysis of prospective studies," *Sleep.* 2010 May;33(5):585-92.

Tamakoshi A, Ohno,"Self-reported sleep duration as a predictor of all-cause mortality: results from the JACC study, Japan," *Sleep.* 2004;27:51–4.

Gallicchio L, Kalesan B, "Sleep duration and mortality: a systematic review and meta-analysis," *J Sleep Res.* 2009;18:148–58.

Knutson KL, Van CE, Rathouz PJ, et al, "Association between sleep and blood pressure in midlife: the CARDIA sleep study," *Arch Intern Med.* 2009;169:1055–61.

Shankar A, Koh WP, Yuan JM, Lee HP, Yu MC, "Sleep duration and coronary heart disease mortality among Chinese adults in Singapore: a population-based cohort study," *Am J Epidemiol.* 2008;168:1367–73.

King CR, Knutson KL, Rathouz PJ, Sidney S, Liu K, Lauderdale DS, "Short sleep duration and incident coronary artery calcification," *JAMA.* 2008;300:2859–66.

Gottlieb DJ, Redline S, Nieto FJ, et al, "Association of usual sleep duration with hypertension: The Sleep Heart Health Study," *Sleep.* 2006;29:1009–14.

Gangwisch JE, Malaspina D, Boden-Albala B, Heymsfield SB, "Inadequate sleep as a risk factor for obesity: analyses of the NHANES I," *Sleep.* 2005;28:1289–96.

Patel SR, Malhotra A, White DP, Gottlieb DJ, Hu FB, "Association between reduced sleep and weight gain in women," *Am J Epidemiol.* 2006;164:947–54.

Patel SR, Hu FB, "Short sleep duration and weight gain: a systematic review," *Obesity.* 2008;16:643–653.

Kaneita Y, Uchiyama M, Yoshiike N, Ohida T, "Associations of usual sleep duration with serum lipid and lipoprotein levels," *Sleep.* 2008;31:645–52.

Stranges S, Dorn JM, Cappuccio FP, et al, "A population-based study of short sleep duration and hypertension: the strongest association may be in pre-menopausal women," *Circulation.* 2009;119:e309.

Stang A, Moebus S, Mohlenkamp S, Erbel R, "Gender-specific associations of short sleep duration with prevalent hypertension," *Hypertension.* 2008;51:e15–e16.

Cappuccio FP, Taggart FM, Kandala N-B, et al, "Meta-analysis of short sleep duration and obesity in children, adolescents and adults," *Sleep.* 2008;31:619–26.

Steptoe A, Peacey V, Wardle J, "Sleep duration and health in young adults," *Arch Intern Med.* 2006;166:1689–92.

Knutson KL, Turek FW, "The U-shaped association between sleep and health: the 2 peaks do not mean the same thing," *Sleep.* 2006;29:878–79.

Patel SR, Ayas NT, Malhotra MR, et al, "A prospective study of sleep duration and mortality risk in women," *Sleep.* 2004;27:440–4.

Hublin C, Partinen M, Koskenvuo M, Kaprio J, "Sleep and mortality: a population-based 22-year follow-up study," *Sleep.* 2007;30:1245–53.

Spiegel K, Tasali E, Leproult R, Van Cauter E, "Effects of poor and short sleep on glucose metabolism and obesity risk," *Nat Rev Endocrinol.* 2009;5:253–61.

Ikehara S, Iso H, Date C, et al, "Association of sleep duration with mortality from cardiovascular disease and other causes for Japanese men and women: the JACC study," *Sleep.* 2009;32:295–301.

Habit 27: Allergy-Proof Yourself and Your Environment

Pelucchi C, Negri E, Gallus S, Boffetta P, Tramacere I, La Vecchia C, "Long-term particulate matter exposure and mortality: a review of European epidemiological studies," *BMC Public Health.* 2009 Dec 8;9:453.

Chen H1, Goldberg MS, Villeneuve PJ, "A systematic review of the relation between long-term exposure to ambient air pollution and chronic diseases," *Rev Environ Health*. 2008 Oct-Dec;23(4):243-97.

Miller KA, Siscovick DS, Sheppard L, Shepherd K, et al, "Long-Term Exposure to Air Pollution and Incidence of Cardiovascular Events in Women," *N Engl J Med*. 2007;356:447-458.

Qiu H, Tian L, Ho KF, Pun VC, Wang X, Yu IT, "Air pollution and mortality: Effect modification by personal characteristics and specific cause of death in a case-only study," *Environ Pollut*. 2015 Feb 9;199C:192-197.

Chang CC1, Chen PS, Yang CY, "Short-term effects of fine particulate air pollution on hospital admissions for cardiovascular diseases: a case-crossover study in a tropical city," *J Toxicol Environ Health A*. 2015;78(4):267-77.

Pope CA, Burnett RT, Thun MJ, Calle EE, Krewski D, Ito K, Thurston GD, "Lung cancer, cardiopulmonary mortality, and long-term exposure to fine particulate air pollution," *JAMA*. 2002;287(9):1132–1141.

Brook RD, Rajagopalan S, Pope CA, Brook JR, Bhatnagar A, Diez-Roux AV, Holguin F, Hong Y, Luepker RV, Mittleman MA, Peters A, Siscovick D, Smith SC, Whitsel L, Kaufman JD, "Particulate matter air pollution and cardiovascular disease: an update to the scientific statement from the American heart association," *Circulation*. 2010;121:2331–2378.

Peters A, Ruckerl R, Cyrys J, "Lessons from air pollution epidemiology for studies of engineered nanomaterials," *J Occup Environ Med*. 2011;53(6 Suppl):S8–S13.

Ruckerl R, Schneider A, Breitner S, Cyrys J, Peters A, "Health effects of particulate air pollution: a review of epidemiological evidence," *Inhal Toxicol*. 2011;23:555–592.

Brunekreef B, Forsberg B, "Epidemiological evidence of effects of coarse airborne particles on health," *Eur Respir J*. 2005;26:309–318.

Laden F, Schwartz J, Speizer FE, Dockery DW, "Reduction in fine particulate Air pollution and mortality: extended follow-up of the Harvard Six cities study," *Am J Respir Crit Care Med*. 2006;173:667–672.

Lepeule J, Laden F, Dockery D, Schwartz J, "Chronic exposure to fine particles and mortality: an extended follow-up of the Harvard six cities study from 1974 to 2009," *Environ Health Perspect*. 2012;120:965–970.

Bell ML, Ebisu K, Peng RD, Samet JM, Dominici F, "Hospital admissions and chemical composition of fine particle air pollution," *Am J Respir Crit Care Med*. 2009;179:1115–1120.

Zanobetti A, Bind MA, Schwartz J, "Particulate air pollution and survival in a COPD cohort," *Environ Health*. 2008;7:48.

Zanobetti A, Schwartz J, "Particulate air pollution, progression, and survival after myocardial infarction," *Environ Health Perspect*. 2007;115:769–775.

Naess O, Piro FN, Nafstad P, Smith GD, Leyland AH, "Air pollution, social deprivation, and mortality: a multilevel cohort study," *Epidemiology*. 2007;18(6):686–694.

Clancy L, Goodman P, Sinclair H, Dockery DW, "Effect of air-pollution control on death rates in Dublin, Ireland: an intervention study," *Lancet*. 2002;360(9341):1210–1214.

Elliott P, Shaddick G, Wakefield JC, de Hoogh C, Briggs DJ, "Long-term associations of outdoor air pollution with mortality in Great Britain," *Thorax*. 2007;62(12):1088–1094.

Pope CA, Burnett RT, Thurston GD, Thun MJ, Calle EE, Krewski D, Godleski JJ, "Cardiovascular mortality and long-term exposure to particulate air pollution: epidemiological evidence of general pathophysiological pathways of disease," *Circulation.* 2004;109(1):71–77.

Habit 28: Find Joy

Post SG, "Altuism, happiness, and health: it's good to be good," *Int J Behav Med.* 2005;12(2):66-77.

Tal Ben-Shahar, *Happier: Learn the Secrets to Daily Joy and Lasting Fulfillment.* New York, New York: McGraw-Hill, 2007.

Seligman M, *Authentic Happiness: Using the New Positive Psychology to Realize Your Potential for Lasting Fulfillment.* New York, New York: Arista Books, 2002.

Frankl V, *Man's Search for Meaning.* New York, New York: Simon & Schuster, 1984.

Lyubomirsky, S, *The How of Happiness: A New Approach to Getting the Life You Want.* New York, New York: Penguin Books, 2008.

Rubin G, *The Happiness Project: Or, Why I Spent a Year Trying to Sing in the Morning, Clean My Closets, Fight Right, Read Aristotle, and Generally Have More Fun.* New York, New York: Harper Collins, 2009.

Berk LS, Tan L, Tan S, "Mirthful laughter, as adjunct therapy in diabetic care, attenuates catecholamines, inflammatory cytokines, CRP, and myocardial infarction occurrence," *The FASEB Journal.* 2008;22:1226.2.

Sabatini F, "The relationship between happiness and health: evidence from Italy," *Soc Sci Med.* 2014 Aug;114:178-87.

Diener E, "Subjective well-being: The science of happiness and a proposal of a national index," *American Psychologist.* 2000;55:34–43.

Diener E, Seligman MEP, "Very happy people," *Psychological Science.* 2002;13:81–84.

Emmons RA, Crumpler CA, "Gratitude as human strength: Appraising the evidence," *Journal of Social and Clinical Psychology.* 2000;19:849–857.

Fredrickson BL, Branigan CA, "Positive emotions broaden scope of attention and thought-action repertoires," *Cognition and Emotion.* 2005;19:313–332.

Fredrickson BL, Joiner T, "Positive emotions trigger upward spirals toward emotional well-being," *Psychological Science.* 2002;13:172–175.

Lyubomirsky S, "Why are some people happier than others?" *American Psychologist.* 2001;56:239–249.

Lyubomirsky S, Tucker KL, Kasri F, "Responses to hedonic conflicting social comparisons: Comparing happy and unhappy people," *European Journal of Social Psychology.* 2001;31:511–535.

McCullough ME, Emmons RA, Tsang J, "The grateful disposition: A conceptual and empirical topography," *Journal of Personality and Social Psychology.* 2002;82:112–127.

Miller M, Fry WF, "The effect of mirthful laughter on the human cardiovascular system," *Med Hypotheses.* 2009 Nov;73(5):636-9.

Park N, Peterson C, Seligman M, "Strengths of character and well-being," *Journal of Social and Clinical Psychology.* 2004;23:603–619.

Seligman M, "Positive psychology: Fundamental assumptions," *Psychologist.* 2003;16:126–127.

Habit 29: Practice Hobbies

Saihara K, Hamasaki S, Ishida S, Kataoka T, Yoshikawa A, Orihara K, et al, "Enjoying hobbies is related to desirable cardiovascular effects," *Heart Vessels*. 2010 Mar;25(2):113-20.

Petersen RC, Doody R, Kurz A, et al, "Current concepts in mild cognitive impairment," *Arch Neurol*. 2001;58(12):1985–1992.

Wilson RS, Mendes De Leon CF, Barnes LL, et al, "Participation in cognitively stimulating activities and risk of incident Alzheimer disease," *JAMA*. 2002;287(6):742–748.

Lisspers J, Sundin O, Ohman A, Hofman-Bang C, Rydén L, Nygren A, "Long-term effects of lifestyle behavior change in coronary artery disease: effects on recurrent coronary events after percutaneous coronary intervention," *Health Psychol*. 2008;24:41–48.

Suwaidi JA, Hamasaki S, Higano ST, Nishimura RA, Holmes DR Jr, Lerman A, "Long-term follow-up of patients with mild coronary artery disease and endothelial dysfunction," *Circulation*. 2000;101:948–954.

Konlaan BB, Bygren LO, Johansson SE, "Visiting the cinema, concerts, museums or art exhibitions as determinant of survival: a Swedish fourteen-year cohort follow-up," *Scand J Public Health*. 2000;28:174–178.

Takahashi T, Matsushita H, "Long-term effects of music therapy on elderly with moderate/severe dementia," *J Music Ther*. 2006;43:317–333.

Giltay EJ, Kamphuis MH, Kalmijn S, Zitman FG, Kromhout D, "Dispositional optimism and the risk of cardiovascular death: the Zutphen Elderly Study," *Arch Intern Med*. 2006;166:431–436.

Al-Khalili F, Janszky I, Andersson A, Svane B, Schenck-Gustafsson K, "Physical activity and performance predict long-term prognosis in middle-aged women surviving acute coronary syndrome," *J Intern Med*. 2007;261:178–187.

Habit 30: Simplify Your Life

Kustenmacher T, Seiwert L, *How To Simplify Your Live: Seven Practical Steps To Letting Go of Your Burdens and Living a Happier Life*. New York, New York: McGraw-Hill, 2004.

Schwartz B, *The Paradox of Choice: Why More is Less*. New York, New York: Harper Collins, 2005.

Ahmed S, "Addiction as a compulsive reward prediction," *Science*. 2004;300:1901–1902.

Camille N, Coricelli G, Sallet J, Pradat P, et al, "The involvement of the orbitofrontal cortex in the experience of regret," *Science*. 2004;304:1167–1170.

Coricelli G, Critchley H, Joffily M, O'Doherty L, Sirigu A, Dolan R, "Regret and its avoidance: a neuroimaging study of choice behavior," *Nat. Neurosci*. 2005;8:1255–1262.

Holt C., Laury S, "Risk aversion and incentive effects," *Am. Econ. Rev.* 2002;92:1644–1655.

McClure S, Laibson D, Loewenstein G, Cohen J, "Separate neural systems value and delayed monetary rewards," *Science*. 2004;306:503–507.

Nozick R, *The Nature of Rationality*. Princeton, NJ: Princeton University Press, 1993.

Persaud N, "Post-decision wagering objectively measures awareness," *Nat. Neurosci*. 2007;10:257–261.

Redish D, "Addiction as a computational process gone awry," *Science*. 2004;306:1944–1947.

Habit 31: Take a Break

Muller W, *Sabbath: Finding Rest, Renewal, and Delight in Our Busy Lives*. New York, New York: Bantam, 2000.

Braun V, Clarke V, "Using thematic analysis in psychology," *Qualitative Research in Psychology*. 2006;3:77–101.

Dein S, "Ritual: The forgotten dimension in mental health," *Psyche and Geloof*. 2011;22(2):91–101.

Heschel A, *Sabbath*. New York, New York: Shambhala, 2003.

Goldberg A, "The Sabbath as dialectic: Implications for mental health," *Journal of Religion and Health*. 1986;25:237–244.

Koenig H, King D, Carson V, *Handbook of religion and health*. New York, New York: Oxford University Press, 2012.

Koenig HG, McCullough ME, Larson D, *Handbook of religion and health*. New York, New York: Oxford University Press, 2001.

Kushner H, *Who needs god?* New York, New York: Summit Books, 1989.

Pargament K, *Spiritually integrated psychotherapy: Understanding and addressing the sacred*. New York, New York: The Guilford Press, 2007.

Poloma MM, Hoelter LF, "The 'Toronto blessing': A holistic model of healing," *Journal for the Scientific Study of Religion*. 1998;37:257–272.

Schumaker J, *Religion and Mental Health*. New York, New York: Oxford University Press, 1992.

Habit 32: Read Every Day

Clare L, Woods B, "A role for cognitive rehabilitation in dementia care," *Neuropsychol Rehabilitation*. 2001;11:193-196.

Hofmann M, Hock C, Kuhler A, Muller-Spahn F, "Interactive computer-based cognitive training in patients with Alzheimer's disease," *J Psychiatr Res*.1996;30:493-501.

Kesslak JP, Nicloul K, Sandman C, "Memory training for individuals with Alzheimer's disease improves name recall," *Alzheimer's Res*. 1997;3:151-157.

Moore S, Sandman CA, McGrady K, Kesslak JP, "Memory training improves cognitive ability in patients with dementia," *Neuropsychol Rehabilitation*. 2001;11:245-261.

Roland PE, *Brain Activation*. New York, New York: Wiley-Liss, 1993.

Price CJ, Wise RJ, Watson JD, Patterson K, Howard D, Frackowiak RS, "Brain activity during reading. The effects of exposure duration and task," *Brain*.1994;117:1255-1269.

Miura N, Iwata K, Watanabe J, Sugiura M, Akitsuki Y, Sassa Y, et al, "Cortical activation during reading aloud of long sentences: fMRI study," *Neuroreport*. 2003;14:1563-1566.

Kreiner DS, Ryan JJ, "Memory and motor skill components of the WAIS-III Digit Symbol-Coding subtest," *Clin Neuropsychol*. 2001;15:109–113.

Miura N, Watanabe J, Iwata K, Sassa Y, Riera J, Tsuchiya H, Sato S, Horie K,

Kawashima R, "Cortical activation during reading of ancient versus modern Japanese texts: fMRI study," *Neuroimage.* 2005;26:426–431.

Ritchie K, Artero S, Touchon J, "Classification criteria for mild cognitive impairment: a population-based validation study," *Neurol.* 2001;56:37–42.

Social

Habit 33: Volunteer Each Week

Harris AH, Thoresen CE, "Volunteering Is Associated With Delayed Mortality In Older People: Analysis of The Longitudinal Study of Aging," *J Health Psychol.* 2005 Nov;10(6):739-52.

Sneed RS, Cohen S, "A Prospective Study of Volunteerism and Hypertension Risk in Older Adults," *Psychology and Aging.* 2013 Jun; Vol 28(2): 578-586.

Brown SL, Brown RM, House JS, Smith DM, "Coping with spousal loss: Potential buffering effects of self-reported helping behavior," *Personality and Social Psychology Bulletin.* 2008;34:849–861.

Konrath S, Fuhrel-Forbis A, Lou A, Brown S, "Motives for volunteering are associated with mortality risk in older adults," *Health Psychol.* 2012;31:87–96.

Von Bonsdorff MB, Rantanen T, "Benefits of formal voluntary work among older people. A review," *Aging Clin Exp Res.* 2011;23:162–169.

Dickens AP, Richards SH, Greaves CJ, Campbell JL, "Interventions targeting social isolation in older people: a systematic review," *BMC Publ Health.* 2011;11:647.

Miller G, Ayalon L, "Volunteering as a predictor of all-cause mortality: what aspects of volunteering really matter?" *Int Psychogeriatr.* 2008;20:1000–1013.

Choi NG, Kim J, "The effect of time volunteering and charitable donations in later life on psychological wellbeing," *Ageing Soc.* 2011;31:590–610.

Luks A, Payne P, *The Healing Power of Doing Good.* iUniverse.com: Lincoln, Nebraska, 1991.

Lum TY, Lightfoot E, "The Effects of Volunteering on the Physical and Mental Health of Older People," *Research on Aging.* 2005;27:31–55.

Kim J, Pai M, "Volunteering and trajectories of depression," *J Aging Health.* 2010;22:84–105.

Li Y, Ferraro KF, "Volunteering and depression in later life: social benefit or selection processes?" *J Health Soc Behav.* 2005;46:68–84.

Morrow-Howell N, Hinterlong J, Rozario PA, Tang F, "Effects of volunteering on the well-being of older adults," *J Gerontol B Psychol Sci Soc Sci.* 2003;58:S137–S145.

Musick MA, Wilson J, "Volunteering and depression: the role of psychological and social resources in different age groups," *Soc Sci Med.* 2003;56:259–269.

Okun MA, August KJ, Rook KS, Newsom JT, "Does volunteering moderate the relation between functional limitations and mortality?" *Soc Sci Med.* 2010;71:1662–1668.

Piliavin JA, Siegl E, "Health benefits of volunteering in the Wisconsin longitudinal study," *J Health Soc Behav.* 2007;48:450–464.

Van Willigen M, "Differential benefits of volunteering across the life course," *J Gerontol B Psychol Sci Soc Sci.* 2000;55:S308–S318.

Li Y, Ferraro KF, "Volunteering in middle and later life: is health a benefit, barrier or both?" *Soc Forces.* 2006;85:497–519.

Morrow-Howell N, Hinterlong J, Rozario PA, Tang F, "Effects of Volunteering on the Well-Being of Older Adults," *Journals of Gerontology: Series B.* 2003;58:S137–S145.

Greenfield EA, Marks NF, "Formal Volunteering as a Protective Factor for Older Adults' Psychological Well-Being," *The Journals of Gerontology, Series B.* 2004;59:S258–S264.

Habit 34: Love Yourself

Peck MS, *The Road Less Travelled.* New York, New York. Touchstone, 1978.

Branden N, *The Six Pillars of Self-Esteem.* New York, New York: Bantam Books, 1994.

Wang F, Veugelers PJ, "Self-esteem and cognitive development in the era of the childhood obesity epidemic," *Obes Rev.* 2008;9(6):615–623.

Mann M, Hosman CM, Schaalma HP, de Vries NK, "Self-esteem in a broad-spectrum approach for mental health promotion," *Health Educ Res.* 2004;19(4):357–372.

Bosacki S, Dane A, Marini Z, "Peer relationships and internalizing problems in adolescents: mediating role of self-esteem," *Emotional and Behavioural Difficulties.* 2007;12(4):261–282.

Strauss RS, "Childhood obesity and self-esteem," *Pediatrics.* 2000;105(1):e15.

Neumark-Sztainer DR, Wall MM, Haines JI, Story MT, Sherwood NE, van den Berg PA, "Shared risk and protective factors for overweight and disordered eating in adolescents," *Am J Prev Med.* 2007;33(5):359–369.

Spencer JM, Zimet GD, Aalsma MC, Orr DP, "Self-esteem as a predictor of initiation of coitus in early adolescents," *Pediatrics.* 2002;109(4):581–584.

Waddell GR, "Labor-Market Consequences of Poor Attitude and Low Self-Esteem in Youth," *Economic Inquiry.* 2006;44(1):69–97.

French S, Story M, Perry C, "Self-esteem and obesity in children and adolescents: a literature review," *Obes Res.* 1995;3:479–490.

Franklin J, Denyer G, Steinbeck KS, Caterson ID, Hill AJ, "Obesity and Risk of Low Self-esteem: A Statewide Survey of Australian Children," *Pediatrics.* 2006;118(6):2481–2487.

Swallen KC, Reither EN, Haas SA, Meier AM, "Overweight, obesity, and health-related quality of life among adolescents: the National Longitudinal Study of Adolescent Health," *Pediatrics.* 2005;115(2):340–347.

O'Dea JA, "Self-concept, self-esteem and body weight in adolescent females: a three-year longitudinal study," *J Health Psychol.* 2006;11(4):599–611.

Habit 35: Love Your Spouse or Partner

Lerner H, *The Dance of Intimacy.* New York, New York: Harper Collins, 1989.

Goleman D, *Emotional Intelligence: Why It Can Matter More Than IQ.* New York, New York: Bantam Books, 1997.

Gottman J, Silver N, *The Seven Principles for Making Marriage Work: A Practical Guide from the Country's Foremost Relationship Expert.* New York, New York: Random House, 2015.

Ornish D, *Love and Survival: The Scientific Basis For The Healing Power of Intimacy.* New York, New York: Harper Collins, 1998.

Umberson Debra, Williams Kristi, Powers Daniel A, Liu Hui, Needham Belinda, "You

Make Me Sick: Marital Quality and Health over the Life Course," *Journal of Health and Social Behavior.* 2006;47:1–16.

Robles Theodore F, Kiecolt-Glaser Janice K, "The Physiology of Marriage: Pathways to Health," *Physiology and Behavior.* 2003;79:409–16.

House JS, Landis KR, Umberson D, "Social relationships and health," *Science.* 1988;241:540–545.

Johnson NJ, Backlund E, Sorlie PD, Loveless CA, "Marital status and mortality: The National Longitudinal Mortality Study," *Ann Epidemiol.* 2000;10:224–238.

Ross CE, Mirowsky J, Goldsteen K, "The impact of the family on health: the decade in review," *J Marriage Fam.* 1990;52:1059–1078.

Umberson D, "Gender, marital status and the social control of health behavior," *Soc Sci Med.* 1992;34:907–917.

Gottman, J, *Why Marriages Succeed or Fail and How You Can Make Yours Last.* New York, New York: Simon & Schuster, 1994.

Robels TF, Kiecolt-Glaser JK, "The physiology of marriage: pathways to health," *Physiol Behav.* 2003;79:409–416.

Christakis Nicholas A, Allison Paul D, "Mortality after the Hospitalization of a Spouse," *The New England Journal of Medicine.* 2006;354:719–30.

Habit 36: Love Your Children

Severe S, *How to Behave So Your Children Will, Too.* New York, New York. Penguin Books, 2003.

Galinsky E, *Mind In The Making: The Seven Essential Life Skills Every Child Needs.* New York, New York: Harper Collins, 2010.

Mogel W, *The Blessing of A Skinned Knee.* New York, New York. Penguin Compass, 2001.

Rosemond J, *The Well-Behaved Child: Discipline That Really Works.* Nashville, Tennessee. Thomas Nelson, 2009.

Eberly S, *365 Manners Kids Should Know.* New York, New York: Three Rivers Press, 2001.

Gordon T, *Parent Effectiveness Training: The Proven Program for Raising Responsible Children.* New York, New York: Three Rivers Press, 2000.

Baker J, *No More Meltdowns: Positive Strategies For Managing and Preventing Out-Of-Control Behavior.* Arlington, Texas: Future Horizons, 2008.

Healy JM, *Endangered Minds: Why Children Don't Think and What We Can Do About It.* New York, New York: Simon & Schuster, 1990.

Winn M, *The Plug-In Drug: Television, Computers, and Family Life.* New York, New York: Penguin Books, 2002.

Boteach S, *Ten Conversations You Need To Have With Your Children.* New York, New York: Harper Collins, 2006.

Dosick W, *Golden Rules: The Ten Ethical Values Parents Need to Teach Their Children.* San Francisco, California: Harper Collins, 1995.

Rolfe R, *The Seven Secrets of Successful Parents.* Chicago, Illinois: Contemporary Books, 1997.

Phelan TW, *1-2-3 Magic: Effective Discipline For Children.* Glen Ellyn, Illinois: Child Management, Inc., 1995.

Walsh D, *No: Why Kids of All Ages Need To Hear It and Ways Parents Can Say It.* New York, New York: Simon & Schuster, 2007.

MacKenzie RJ, *Setting Limits: How To Raise Responsible, Independent Children By Providing Clear Boundaries.* New York, New York: Random House, 1998.

Galinsky E, *Mind in the Making: The Seven Essential Life Skills Every Child Needs.* Harper Collins: New York, New York, 2010.

Siegel DJ, Bryson TP, *The Whole-Brain Child: 12 Revolutionary Strategies to Nurture Your Child's Developing Mind.* New York, New York: Random House, 2011.

Nerburn K, *Letters to My Son: A Father's Wisdom on Manhood, Life, and Love.* Novato, California: New World Library, 1999.

Covey SR, *The 7 Habits of Highly Effective Families.* New York, New York: Golden Books, 1997.

Faber A, Mazlish E, *How to Talk So Kids Will Listen & Listen So Kids Will Talk.* Avon Books: New York, New York: Scribner, 1980.

Bernstein J, *10 Days To A Less Defiant Child: The Breakthrough Program For Overcoming Your Child's Difficult Behavior.* New York, New York: Marlowe & Company, 2006.

Radcliffe SC, *Raise Your Kids Without Raising Your Voice.* New York, New York: BPS Books, 2006.

Brooks R, Goldstein S, *Raising Resilient Children. Raising Resilient Children: Fostering Strength, Hope, and Optimism in Your Child.* New York, New York: McGraw-Hill, 2001.

Rosenberg M, *Nonviolent Communication: A Language of Life.* New York, New York: Puddle Dancer Press, 2003.

Kurcinka MS, *Kids, Parents, and Power Struggles: Winning For A Lifetime.* New York, New York: Harper Collins, 2000.

DeVore ER, Ginsburg KR, "The protective effects of good parenting on adolescents," *Curr Opin Pediatr.* 2005 Aug;17(4):460-5.

Fletcher AC, Steinberg L, Williams-Wheeler M, "Parental influences on adolescent problem behavior: revisiting Stattin and Kerr," *Child Dev.* 2004;75:781-796.

Habit 37: Love Your Friends & Family

Feiler B, *The Secrets of Happy Families: Improve Your Mornings, Tell Your Family History, Fight Smarter, Go Out and Play, and Much More.* New York, New York: Harper Collins, 2013.

Biddulph S, *The Secret of Happy Children: Why Children Behave The Way They Do and What You Can Do To Help Them To Be Optimistic, Loving, Capable, and Happy.* New York, New York: Marlowe & Company, 2002

Williams V, Williams R, *Life Skills: Eight Simple Ways to Build Stronger Relationships, Communicate More Clearly, and Improve Your Health.* New York, New York: Random Health, 1997.

Ricker A, *How Happy Families Happen: Six Steps To Bringing Emotional and Spiritual Health Into Your Home.* Center City, Minnesota: Hazelden Foundation, 2006.

Umberson D, Montez JK, "Social relationships and health: a flashpoint for health policy," *J Health Soc Behav.* 2010;51 (Suppl):S54-66.

Pennebaker JW, *Opening Up: The Healing Power of Expressing Emotions.* The Guilford Press: New York, New York, 1997.

Antonovsky A, *Unraveling the Mystery of Health.* San Francisco, CA: Jossey-Bass, 1987.

Cacioppo JT, Hawkley LC, Elizabeth CL, Ernst JM, Burleson MH, Kowalewski RB, Malarkey WB, Van Cauter E, Berntson GG, "Loneliness and Health: Potential Mechanisms," *Psychosomatic Medicine.* 2002;64:407–17.

Christakis NA, Fowler JH, "The Spread of Obesity in a Large Social Network over 32 Years," *The New England Journal of Medicine*. 2007;357:370–79.

Cohen S, "Social Relationships and Health," *American Psychologist*. 2004;59:676–84.

Crosnoe R, Elder GH, "From Childhood to the Later Years: Pathways of Human Development," *Research on Aging*. 2004;26:623–54.

Uchino BN, *Social Support and Physical Health: Understanding the Health Consequences of Relationships*. New Haven, CT: Yale University Press, 2004.

Habit 38: Participate in Your Community

Covey SM, *The Speed of Trust: The One Thing That Changes Everything*. New York, New York: Simon & Schuster, 2006.

LeCompte A, *Creating Harmonious Relationships: A Practical Guide To The Power of True Empathy*. Portsmouth, New Hampshire: Atlantic Books, 2000.

Rodriguez-Artalejo F, Guallar-Castillon P, Herrera MC, et al, "Social network as a predictor of hospital readmission and mortality among older patients with heart failure," *J Card Fail*. 2006;12(8):621-627.

Brownstein JN, Chowdhury FM, Norris SL, et al, "Effectiveness of community health workers in the care of people with hypertension," *Am J Prev Med*. 2007;32(5):435-447.

Berthold TA, Miller J, Avila-Esparza A, *Foundations for Community Health Workers*. San Francisco, CA: John Wiley & Sons, Inc., 2009.

MacGregor K, Wong S, Sharifi C, Handley M, Bodenheimer T, "The action plan project: discussing behavior change in the primary care visit," *Ann Fam Med*. 2005;3(Suppl 2):S39-S40.

Hibbard JH, Stockard J, Mahoney ER, Tusler M, "Development of the Patient Activation Measure (PAM): conceptualizing and measuring activation in patients and consumers," *Health Serv Res*. 2004;39(4, pt 1):1005-1026.

Mitchell PH, Powell L, Blumenthal J, et al, "A short social support measure for patients recovering from myocardial infarction: the ENRICHD Social Support Inventory," *J Cardiopulm Rehabil*. 2003;23(6):398-403.

Habit 39: Find Mentors

Ramanan RA, Taylor WC, Davis RB, Phillips RS, "Mentoring matters. Mentoring and career preparation in internal medicine residency training," *J Gen Intern Med*. 2006 Apr;21(4):340-5.

Kogan SM, Brody GH, Chen YF, "Natural mentoring processes deter externalizing problems among rural African American emerging adults: a prospective analysis," *Am J Community Psychol*. 2011 Dec;48(3-4):272-83.

Stewart C, Openshaw L, "Youth mentoring: what is it and what do we know?" *J Evid Based Soc Work*. 2014;11(4):328-36.

Balmer D, D'Alessandro D, Risko W, Gusic ME, "How mentoring relationships evolve: a longitudinal study of academic pediatricians in a physician educator faculty development program," *J Contin Educ Health Prof*. 2011 Spring;31(2):81-6.

Larsen E, *Destination Joy: Moving Beyond Fear, Loss, and Trauma in Recover*. Center City, Minnesota: Hazelden Foundation, 2010.

Dorsey LE, Baker CM, "Mentoring undergraduate nursing students," *Nurse Educator*. 2004;29:260-265.

DuBois DL, Holloway BE, Valentine JC, Cooper H, "Effectiveness of mentoring programs for youth: A meta-analytic review," *American Journal of Community Psychology.* 2002;30:157-197.

DuBois DL, Karcher MA, editors, *Handbook of youth mentoring.* Thousand Oaks, CA: Sage, 2005.

DuBois DL, Silverthorn N, "Natural mentoring relationships and adolescent health: Evidence from a national study," *American Journal of Public Health.* 2005;95:518–524.

Ng TWH, Eby LT, Sorensen KL, Feldman DC, "Predictors of objective and subjective career success: A meta-analysis," *Personnel Psychology.* 2005;58:367–408.

Rhodes JE, *Stand by me: The risks and rewards of mentoring today's youth.* Cambridge, MA: Harvard University Press, 2002.

Rhodes JE, Grossman JB, Rensch NR, "Agents of change: Pathways through which mentoring relationships influence adolescent's academic adjustment," *Child Development.* 2000;71:1662–1671.

Spirituality and Values

Habit 40: Live Your Values

Ornish D, *Love and Survival: The Scientific Basis For The Healing Power of Intimacy.* New York, New York: Harper Collins, 1998.

Covey SR, *The 7 Habits of Highly Effective People.* New York, New York: Simon & Schuster, 1989.

Ruiz DM, *The Four Agreements: A Practical Guide to Personal Freedom.* San Rafael, California: Amber-Allen Publishing, 1997.

Habit 41: Practice Your Faith or Spiritual Practice

Benson H, Stark M. *Timeless Healing: The Power and Biology of Belief.* New York, New York: Simon & Schuster, 1996.

Koenig HG, *The Healing Power of Faith: Science Explores Medicine's Last Great Frontier.* New York, New York: Simon & Schuster, 1999.

Levin J, *God, Faith, and Health: Exploring The Spirituality-Healing Connection.* Danvers, Massachusetts: John Wiley & Sons, 2001.

Kornfield J, *After The Ecstasy, The Laundry: How The Heart Grows Wise on The Spiritual Path.* New York, New York: Bantam Books, 2000.

Matthews DA, Clark C, *The Faith Factor: Proof of The Healing Power of Prayer.* New York, New York: Penguin Books, 1999.

Yoshimoto SM, Ghorbani S, Baer JM, et al, "Religious coping and problem-solving by couples faced with prostate cancer," *European Journal of Cancer Care.* 2006;15(5):481–488.

Shaw B, Han JY, Kim E, et al, "Effects of prayer and religious expression within computer support groups on women with breast cancer," *Psycho-Oncology.* 2007;16(7):676–687.

Cooper-Effa M, Blount W, Kaslow N, Rothenberg R, Eckman J, "Role of spirituality in patients with sickle cell disease," *Journal of the American Board of Family Practice.* 2001;14(2):116–122.

Giaquinto S, Spiridigliozzi C, Caracciolo B, "Can faith protect from emotional distress after stroke?" *Stroke.* 2007;38(3):993–997.

Rinaldi S, Ghisi M, Iaccarino L, et al, "Influence of coping skills on health-related quality of life in patients with systemic lupus erythematosus," *Arthritis Care and Research.* 2006;55(3):427–433.

Tepper L, Rogers SA, Coleman EM, Malony HN, "The prevalence of religious coping among persons with persistent mental illness," *Psychiatric Services.* 2001;52(5):660–665.

Brown SL, Nesse RM, House JS, Utz RL, "Religion and emotional compensation: results from a prospective study of widowhood," *Personality and Social Psychology Bulletin.* 2004;30(9):1165–1174.

Idler EL, Kasl SV, Hays JC, "Patterns of religious practice and belief in the last year of life," *Journals of Gerontology B.* 2001;56(6):S326–S334.

Scholte WF, Olff M, Ventevogel P, et al, "Mental health symptoms following war and repression in Eastern Afghanistan," *Journal of the American Medical Association.* 2004;292(5):585–593.

Schuster MA, Stein BD, Jaycox LH, et al, "A national survey of stress reactions after the September 11, 2001, terrorist attacks," *New England Journal of Medicine.* 2001;345(20):1507–1512.

Krause N, "Religious meaning and subjective well-being in late life," *J Gerontol B Psychol Sci Soc Sci.* 2003 May;58(3):S160-70.

Krause N, "Religious doubt and psychological well-being: a longitudinal investigation," *Review of Religious Research.* 2006;47(3):287–302.

Habit 42: Let Go of Emotional Pain from the Past

Kubler-Ross E, *On Death and Dying: What the Dying Have to Teach Doctors, Nurses, Clergy and Their Own Families.* New York, New York: Simon & Schuster, 1969.

Higgins GO, *Resilient Adults: Overcoming A Cruel Past.* San Francisco, California: Jossey Bass, 1994.

Callanan M, Kelley P, *Final Gifts: Understanding the Special Awareness, Needs, and Communications of the Dying.* New York, New York: Simon & Schuster, 2012.

Muller W, *Legacy of The Heart: The Spiritual Advantages of A Painful Childhood.* New York, New York: Simon & Schuster, 1992.

Kushner HS, *When Bad Things Happen To Good People.* New York, New York: Schocken Books, 1981.

Herman JL, *Trauma and Recovery.* New York, New York: Harper Collins, 1992.

Knapp C, *Drinking: A Love Story.* New York, New York: Dell Publishing, 1997

Lampert R, Shusterman V, Burg M, McPherson C, et al, "Anger-Induced T-Wave Alternans Predicts Future Ventricular Arrhythmias in Patients With Implantable Cardioverter-Defibrillators," J Am Coll Cardiol. 2009;53:774-778.

Shear MK, Wang Y, Skritskaya N, Duan N, Mauro C, Ghesquiere A, "Treatment of complicated grief in elderly persons: a randomized clinical trial," *JAMA Psychiatry.* 2014 Nov;71(11):1287-95.

Habit 43: Live Within Your Means

Ramsey D, *The Total Money Makeover: Classic Edition: A Proven Plan for Financial Fitness.* Nashville, Tennessee: Harper Collins, 2013.

Kahn JR, Pearlin LI, "Financial strain over the life course and health among older adults," *J Health Soc Behav* 2006; 47:17–31.

Adler NE, Stewart J, "Health disparities across the lifespan: meaning, methods, and mechanisms," *Ann N Y Acad Sci.* 2010;1186:5–23.

Braveman PA, Cubbin C, Egerter S, Chideya S, Marchi KS, Metzler M, et al, "Socioeconomic status in health research: one size does not fit all," *JAMA.* 2005;294:2879–2888.

Bridges S, Disney R, "Debt and depression," *J Health Econ.* 2010;29:388–403.

Dossey L, "Debt and health," *Explore.* 2007;3:83–90.

Drentea P, Reynolds JR, "Neither a Borrower Nor a Lender Be: The Relative Importance of Debt and SES for Mental Health Among Older Adults," *J Aging Health.* 2012;24:673–695.

Fremstad S, Traub A, *Discrediting America: The Urgent Need to Reform the Nation's Credit Reporting Industry.* New York, New York: Demos, 2011.

Garcia J, *Borrowing to Make Ends Meet: The Rapid Growth of Credit Card Debt in America.* New York, New York: Demos, 2007.

Graeber D, *Debt: The First 5,000 Years.* New York, New York: Melville House, 2011.

Gruenstein BD, Wei L, Ernst KS, *Foreclosures by Race and Ethnicity: The Demographics of a Crisis.* Washington, D.C: Center for Responsible Lending, 2010.

Jenkins R, Bhugra D, Bebbington P, Brugha T, Farrell M, Coid J, et al, "Debt, income and mental disorder in the general population," *Psychol Med.* 2008;38:1485–1493.

Matthews KA, Gallo LC, "Psychological perspectives on pathways linking socioeconomic status and physical health," *Annu Rev Psychol.* 2011;62:501–530.

McLaughlin KA, Nandi A, Keyes KM, Uddin M, Aiello AE, Galea S, et al, "Home foreclosure and risk of psychiatric morbidity during the recent financial crisis," *Psychol Med.* 2011:1–8.

Reading R, Reynolds S, "Debt, social disadvantage and maternal depression," *Soc Sci Med.* 2001;53:441–453.

Selenko E, Batinic B, "Beyond debt. A moderator analysis of the relationship between perceived financial strain and mental health," *Soc Sci Med.* 2011;73:1725–1732.

Shavers VL, "Measurement of socioeconomic status in health disparities research," *J Natl Med Assoc.* 2007;99:1013–1023.

Sweet E, "Symbolic capital, consumption, and health inequality," *Am J Public Health.* 2011;101:260– 264.

Habit 44: Practice Integrity

Covey S.R., *The 7 Habits of Highly Effective People.* New York, New York: Simon & Schuster, 1989.

Ruiz DM, *The Four Agreements: A Practical Guide to Personal Freedom.* San Rafael, California: Amber-Allen Publishing, 1997.

Branden N, *Taking Responsibility: Self-Reliance and The Accountable Life.* New York, New York: Simon & Schuster, 1996.

Wood AM, Linley PA, Maltby J, Baliousis, M, Joseph S, "The Authentic Personality: A Theoretical and Empirical Conceptualization and The Development of The Authenticity Scale," *Journal of Counseling Psychology.* Jul 2008; Vol 55(3); 385-399.

Izzo, J, *Stepping Up: How Taking Responsibility Changes Everything.* San Francisco, California: Berrett-Koehler Publishers, 2012.

Telushkin J, *Words That Hurt, Words That Heal: How to Choose Words Wisely and Well.* New York, New York: William Morrow, 1996.

Biro BD, *Beyond Success: The 15 Secrets of a Winning Life*. Hamilton, Montana: Pygmalion Press, 1997.

Habit 45: Leave a Legacy

Newman B, *Leave Your Legacy: The Power to Unleash Your Greatness*. Greenleaf Book. Austin, TX: Group Press, 2015.

Ambrose S, Bridges MW, Lovett MC, DiPietro M, Norman MK, *How Learning Works: Seven Research-Based Principles For Smart Teaching*. San Francisco, California: Jossey-Bass, 2010.

Henry T, *Die Empty: Unleash Your Best Work Every Day*. New York, New York: Random House, 2013.

Zaval L, Markowitz EM, Weber EU, "How will I be remembered? Conserving the environment for the sake of one's legacy," *Psychol Sci*. 2015; 26(2):231-6.

Habit 46: Visualize Before You Act

Casey A, Benson H, MacDonald A, *Mind Your Heart A Mind-Body Approach To Stress Management Exercise And Nutrition For Heart Health*. New York, New York: Simon & Schuster, 2004.

Hammond J, Keeney R, Raiffa H, *Smart Choices: A Practical Guide to Making Better Decisions*. Crown Business: Watertown, Massachusetts: Harvard Business Review Press, 1999.

Gawain S, *Creative Visualization: Use the Power of Your Imagination to Create What You Want in Your Life*. Novato, CA: New World Library, 2002.

Johnson S, *Yes or No: The Guide to Better Decisions*. New York, New York: Harper Collins, 1993.

Barry MJ, Edgman-Levitan S, "Shared decision making–pinnacle of patient-centered care," *New Engl J Med*. 2012;366(9):780–1.

Emanuel EJ, Emanuel LL, "Four models of the physician-patient relationship," *JAMA*. 1992;267:2221.

Charles C, Gafni A, Whelan T, "Shared decision-making in the medical encounter: what does it mean?" *Soc Sci Med*. 1997;44:681–92.

Joyce J, *The Foundations of Causal Decision Theory*. Cambridge, UK: Cambridge University Press, 1999.

Pieters R, Zeelenberg M, "On bad decisions and deciding badly: when intention-behavior inconsistency is regrettable," *Organ. Behav. Hum. Decis. Process*. 2003;97:18–30.

Habit 47: Practice Gratitude: The Secret To Happiness

Emmons RA, *Thanks: How The New Science of Gratitude Can Make You Happier*. New York, New York: Houghton Mifflin, 2007.

Baker D, Stauth C, *What Happy People Know: How The New Science of Happiness Can Change Your Life For The Better*. Emmaus, Pennsylvania: Rodale Books, 2003.

Ray V, *Choosing Happiness: The Art of Living Unconditionally*. Center City, Minnesota: Hazelden Foundation, 1991.

Gilbert, D, *Stumbling on Happiness*. New York, New York: Alred A. Knopf, 2006.

Emmons RA, *Gratitude Works!: A 21-Day Program for Creating Emotional Prosperity.* San Francisco, California: Jossey-Bass, 2013.

Hallowell E, *The Childhood Roots of Adult Happiness: Five Steps to Help Kids Create and Sustain Lifelong Joy.* Toronto, Canada. Ballantine Books, 2003.

Froh JJ, Bono G, *Making Grateful Kids: The Science of Building Character.* West Conshohocken, Pennsylvania: Templeton Press, 2014.

Lambert NM, Graham SM, Fincham FD, "A prototype analysis of gratitude: varieties of gratitude experiences," *Pers Soc Psychol Bull.* 2009;35:1193–1207.

Emmons RA, McCullough ME, editors. *The Psychology of Gratitude.* New York, New York: Oxford University Press, 2004.

Eid M, Larsen RJ, editors. *The Science of Subjective Well-Being.* New York, New York: Guilford Press, 2008.

Dickerhoof RM, "Expressing optimism and gratitude: a longitudinal investigation of cognitive strategies to increase well-being," *Diss Abstr Int.* 2007;68:4174B.

Froh JJ, Sefick WJ, Emmons RA, "Counting blessings in early adolescents: an experimental study of gratitude and subjective well-being," *J Sch Psychol.* 2008;46:213–233.

Wood AM, Joseph S, Maltby J, "Gratitude uniquely predicts satisfaction with life: incremental validity above the domains and facets of the five factor model," *Pers Individ Dif.* 2008;45:49–54.

Chen LH, Kee YH, "Gratitude and adolescent athletes' well-being," *Soc Indic Res.* 2008;89:361–373.

Froh JJ, Yurkewicz C, Kashdan TB, "Gratitude and subjective well-being in early adolescence: examining gender differences," *J Adolesc.* 2009;32:633–650.

Emmons RA, McCullough ME, "Counting blessings versus burdens: an experimental investigation of gratitude and subjective well-being in daily life," *J Pers Soc Psychol.* 2003 Feb;84(2):377-89.

Wood AM, Joseph S, Lloyd J, Atkins S, "Gratitude influences sleep through the mechanism of pre-sleep cognitions," *J Psychosom Res.* 2009;66:43–48.

Polak EL, McCullough ME, "Is gratitude an alternative to materialism?" *J Happiness Stud.* 2006;7:343–360.

Gurel Kirgiz O, "Effects of gratitude on subjective well-being, self-control, and memory," *Diss Abstr Int.* 2008;68:4825B.

Henrie P, "The effects of gratitude on divorce adjustment and well-being of middle-aged divorced women," *Diss Abstr Int.* 2007;67:6096B.

Mallen Ozimkowski K, "The gratitude visit in children and adolescents: an investigation of gratitude and subjective well-being," *Diss Abstr Int.* 2008;69:686B.

Habit 48: The Power of Music

Warth M, Kessler J, Koenig J, Wormit AF, Hillecke TK, Bardenheuer HJ, "Music therapy to promote psychological and physiological relaxation in palliative care patients: protocol of a randomized controlled trial," *BMC Palliat Care.* 2014 Dec 17;13(1):60.

Bradt J, Dileo C, Potvin N, "Music for stress and anxiety reduction in coronary heart disease patients," *Cochrane Database Syst Rev.* 2013 Dec;28:12.

Belgrave M, "The effect of a music therapy intergenerational program on children and older adults' intergenerational interactions, cross-age attitudes, and older adults' psychosocial well-being," *J Music Ther.* 2011;48:486–508.

Eschrich S, Münte TF, Altenmüller EO, "Unforgettable film music: the role of emotion in episodic long-term memory for music," *BMC Neurosci.* 2008;9:48.

Schendel ZA, Palmer C, "Suppression effects on musical and verbal memory," *Mem Cognit.* 2007;35:640–650.

Thoma MV, La Marca R, Bronnimann R, Finkel L, Ehlert U, Nater UM, "The Effect of Music on the Human Stress Response, *PLoS One.* 2013 Aug;5;8(8):e70156.

Ho YC, Cheung MC, Chan AS, "Music training improves verbal but not visual memory: cross-sectional and longitudinal explorations in children," *Neuropsychology.* 2003;17:439–450.

Sluming V, Brooks J, Howard M, Downes JJ, Roberts N, "Broca's area supports enhanced visuospatial cognition in orchestral musicians," *J Neurosci.* 2007;27:3799–3806.

Baumgartner T, Lutz K, Schmidt CF, Jäncke L, "The emotional power of music: how music enhances the feeling of affective pictures," *Brain Res.* 2006;1075:151–164.

Kemper KJ, Danhauer SC, "Music as Therapy," *South Med J.* 2005 Mar;98(3):282-8.

Blood AJ, Zatorre RJ, "Intensely pleasurable responses to music correlate with activity in brain regions implicated in reward and emotion," *Proc Natl Acad Sci USA.* 2001;98:11818–11823.

Samson S, Peretz I, "Effects of prior exposure on music liking and recognition in patients with temporal lobe lesions," *Ann NY Acad Sci.* 2005;1060:419–428.

Simmons-Stern NR, Budson AE, Ally BA, "Music as a Memory Enhancer in Patients with Alzheimer's Disease," *Neuropsychologia.* 2010 Aug; 48(10): 3164–3167.

Cadigan ME, Caruso NA, Haldeman SM, McNamara ME, Noyes DA, et al, "The effects of music on cardiac patients on bed rest," *Progress in Cardiovascular Nursing.* 2001;16(1):5-13.

Chan MF, "Effects of music on patients undergoing a C-clamp procedure after percutaneous coronary interventions: A randomized controlled trial," *Heart & Lung* 2007;36:431-9.

Mandel SE, Hanser SB, Secic M, Davis BA, "Effects of music therapy on health-related outcomes in cardiac rehabilitation: A randomized controlled trial," *Journal of Music Therapy.* 2007;34(3):176-97.

Habit 49: Forgiveness

Luskin F, *Forgive For Good: A Proven Prescription For Health and Happiness.* New York, New York: Harper Collins, 2002.

McMahon S, *Coping With Life's Stressors.* New York, New York: Dell Publishing, 1996.

Schimmel S, *Wounds Not Healed By Time: The Power of Repentance and Forgiveness.* New York, New York: Oxford University Press, 2002.

Lerner H, *The Dance of Anger.* New York, New York: Harper Collins, 1985.

Ruskan J, *Emotional Clearing.* New York, New York: Broadway Books, 2000.

Larsen E, *Destination Joy: Moving Beyond Fear, Loss, & Trauma in Recovery.* Center City, Minnesota: Hazelden Foundation, 2003.

Kushner HS, *Overcoming Life's Disappointments.* New York, New York: Alfred Knopf, 2006.

Wiesenthal S, *The Sunflower: On The Possibilities and Limits of Forgiveness.* New York, New York: Schocken Books, 1997.

Simon S, Simon S, *Forgiveness: How To Make Peace With Your Past and Get On With Your Life.* New York, New York: Warner Books, 1990.

Hallowell EM, *Dare To Forgive*. Deerfield Beach, Florida: Health Communications, 2004.

Smedes LB, *The Art of Forgiving: When You Need To Forgive and Don't Know How*. New York, New York: Random House, 1996.

Toussaint LL, Owen, AD, Cheadle A, "Forgive to live: Forgiveness, health, and longevity," *Journal Of Behavioral Medicine*. 2012;35(4):375-386.

Li, W, Mack D, Enright RD, et al, "Effects of forgiveness therapy on anger, mood, and vulnerability to substance use among inpatient substance-dependent clients," *Journal of Consulting and Clinical Psychology*. 2004;72:1114–1121.

Al-Mubak, RH, Enright RD, "Forgiveness education with parentally love-deprived late adolescents," *J Moral Educ*. 1995;24:427–445.

McCullough MA, Pargament KI, Thoresen CE, *Forgiveness: Theory, Research, and Practice*. New York, New York: The Guilford Press, 2001.

Witvliet CV, Ludwig T, Vander Lann K, "Granting forgiveness or harboring grudges (Implications for emotion, physiology, and health)," *Psychol Sci*. 2001;121:117–123.

Habit 50: Practice Mindfulness

Kabat-Zinn J, *Wherever You Go, There You Are*. New York, New York: Hachette Books, 1994.

Benson H. Stuart EM, *The Wellness Book: The Comprehensive Guide To Maintaining Health and Treating Stress-Related Illness*. New York, New York: Simon & Schuster, 1992.

Langer E, *Mindfulness*. Philadelphia, Pennsylvania: Da Capo Press, 1989.

Tolle E, *The Power of Now: A Guide To Spiritual Enlightenment*. Novato, California: New World Library, 1999.

Branden N, *The Art of Living Consciously: The Power of Awareness To Transform Everyday Life*. New York, New York: Simon & Schuster, 1997.

Gunaratana BH, *Mindfulness In Plain English*. Somerville, Massachusetts: Wisdom Publications, 2011.

"Everyone's Waiting." *Six Feet Under*. HBO. August 21, 2005. Television.

Winner J, *Take The Stress Out of Your Life: A Medical Doctor's Proven Program To Minimize Stress and Maximize Health*. Boston, Massachusetts: Da Capo Press, 2008.

Williams M, Penman D, *Mindfulness: An Eight-Week Plan for Finding Peace in a Frantic World*, Emmaus, Pennsylvania: Rodale Books, 2012.

Duncan S, *Present Moment Awareness: A Simple, Step-By-Step Guide To Living In The Now*. Novato, California. New World Library, 2003

Csikszentmihalyi M, *Finding Flow: The Psychology of Engagement with Everyday Life*. New York, New York: Basic Books, 1998.

Kabat-Zinn J, *Full catastrophic living: Using the wisdom of your body and mind to face stress, pain and illness*. New York, New York: Bantam Dell, 1991.

Carlson LE, Speca M, Patel KD, Goodey E, "Mindfulness-based stress reduction in relation to quality of life, mood, symptoms of stress and immune parameters in breast and prostate cancer outpatients," *Psychosom Med*. 2003;65:571–81.

Bowen S, Witkiewitz K, Dillworth TM, Chawla N, Simpson TL, Ostafin BD, et al, "Mindfulness meditation and substance use in an incarcerated population," *Psychol Addict Behav*. 2006;20:343–7.

Merkes M, "Mindfulness-based stress reduction for people with chronic diseases," *Aust J Prim Health*. 2010;16:200–10.

Fjorback LO, Arendt M, Ornbøl E, Fink P, Walach H, "Mindfulness-based stress reduction and mindfulness-based cognitive therapy - a systematic review of randomized controlled trials," *Acta Psychiatr Scand.* 2011;124:102–19.

Tacon AM, McComb J, Caldera Y, Randolph P, "Mindfulness meditation, anxiety reduction, and heart disease: A pilot study," *Fam Community Health.* 2003;26:25–33.

King MS, Carr T, D'Cruz C, "Transcendental meditation, hypertension and heart disease," *Aust Fam Physician.* 2002;31:164–8.

Paul-Labrador M, Polk D, Dwyer JH, Velasquez I, Nidich S, Rainforth M, et al, "Effects of a randomized controlled trial of transcendental meditation on components of the metabolic syndrome in subjects with coronary heart disease," *Arch Intern Med.* 2006;166:1218–24.

Grossman P, Niemann L, Schmidt S, Walach H, "Mindfulness-based stress reduction and health benefits. A meta-analysis," *J Psychosom Res.* 2004;57:35–43.

Chapter 7

Covey SR, *The 7 Habits of Highly Effective People.* New York, New York: Simon & Schuster, 1989.

Peck MS, *The Road Less Travelled.* New York, New York. Touchstone, 1978.

Table 1

Powerhouse Fruits and Vegetables (N = 41), by Ranking of Nutrient Density Scores[a], 2014			
Nutrient Density Scores			
Food	Score	Food	Score
Watercress	100.00	Scallion	27.35
Chinese cabbage	91.99	Kohlrabi	25.92
Chard	89.27	Cauliflower	25.13
Beet green	87.08	Cabbage	24.51
Spinach	86.43	Carrot	22.6
Chicory	73.36	Tomato	20.37
Leaf lettuce	70.73	Lemon	18.72
Parsley	65.59	Iceberg lettuce	18.28
Romaine lettuce	63.48	Strawberry	17.59
Collard green	62.49	Radish	16.91
Turnip green	62.12	Winter squash (all varieties)	13.89
Mustard green	61.39	Orange	12.91
Endive	60.44	Lime	12.23
Chive	54.80	Grapefruit (pink and red)	11.64
Kale	49.07	Rutabaga	11.58
Dandelion green	46.34	Turnip	11.43
Red pepper	41.26	Blackberry	11.39
Arugula	37.65	Leek	10.69
Broccoli	34.89	Sweet potato	10.51
Pumpkin	33.82	Grapefruit (white)	10.47
Brussels sprout	32.23		

[a] Calculated as the mean of percent daily values (DVs) (based on a 2,000 kcal/d diet) for 17 nutrients (potassium, fiber, protein, calcium, iron, thiamin, riboflavin, niacin, folate, zinc, and vitamins A, B_6, B_{12}, C, D, E, and K) as provided by 100 g of food, expressed per 100 kcal of food. Scores above 100 were capped at 100 (indicating that the food provides, on average, 100% DV of the qualifying nutrients per 100 kcal).

Reproduced from www.cdc.gov

Table 2

Protein Source	Serving Size	Protein/serving
Greek Yogurt	8 oz.	23 g.
Halibut	3 oz.	23 g.
Salmon	3 oz.	23 g.
Chicken	3 oz.	22 g.
Tuna (light)	3 oz.	22 g.
Tilapia	3 oz.	21 g.
Turkey Breast	3 oz.	21 g.
Whey Protein	3 oz.	18 g.
Smoothie Drink	1 cup	16 g.
Cottage Cheese	½ cup	14 g.
Lentils (dried)	¼ cup	13 g.
Soba Noodles	3 oz.	12 g.
Tofu	3 oz.	12 g.
Pinto Beans	½ cup	11 g.
Adzuki Beans	½ cup	9 g.
Edamame	½ cup	9 g.
Black Beans	½ cup	8 g.
Peanut Butter	2 tbsp.	8 g.
Chickpeas	½ cup	7 g.
Green Peas	1 cup	7 g.
Greek Yogurt (frozen)	½ cup	6 g.
Kamut	½ cup	6 g.
Mixed Nuts	2 oz.	6 g.
Quinoa	1 cup	5 g.

Table 3

List of 100 Hobbies

Acting	Gardening	Rafting
Backgammon	Movies	Reading To The Elderly
Badminton	Golf	Renaissance Faire
Basketball	Gymnastics	Rescuing Animals
Bicycling	Hiking	Rock Collecting
Bird watching	Iceskating	Running
Blogging	Jewelry Making	Scrapbooking
Bowling	Jigsaw Puzzles	Scuba Diving
Meals on Wheels driver	Juggling	Sewing
Building Dollhouses	Jump Roping	Skiing
Butterfly Watching	Kayaking	Singing In Choir
Cake Decorating	Kites	Snorkeling
Calligraphy	Knitting	Snowboarding
Camping	Learn Foreign Language	Soccer
Candle Making	Legos	Spend time with family
Canoeing	Lacrosse	Stamp Collecting
Cars	Macramé	Storytelling
Ceramics	Magic	Surfing
Chess	Making Model Cars	Survival
Church/church activities	Martial Arts	Swimming
Coin Collecting	Meditation	Tennis
Collecting Antiques	Modeling Ships	Toy Collecting
Collecting Artwork	Models	Traveling
Collecting Hats	Motorcycles	Tutoring Children
Collecting Sports Cards	Mountain Biking	Ultimate Frisbee
Compose Music	Mountain Climbing	Volunteering
Computer activities	Musical Instruments	Walking
Cooking	Nail Art	Weightlifting
Crochet	Needlepoint	Woodworking
Crossword Puzzles	Painting	Wrestling
Dancing	Photography	Yoga
Fishing	Playing music	Ziplining
Floral Arrangements	Pottery	
Games	Quilting	

Table 4

Volunteer Activity Ideas	
Volunteer at your local library	Give to families of those serving in the military
Visit a nursing home or assisted care facility	Donate blood
Help special needs kids or adults	Do something kind for someone who has suffered a recent loss
Deliver food to those who are unable to leave their home	Donate children's books, novels, and other reading materials to shelters, libraries, and schools
Volunteer at a crisis line	Write a letter to your Congressman about an issue that you care about
Help a family new to town	Offer to rake leaves, shovel the walk, or do housework for an elderly neighbor
Volunteer at a homeless shelter	Teach computer skills to the elderly
Help an adult learn how to read	Become a volunteer tutor
Do something kind for another without being asked	Coach a sport
Volunteer at a local homeless shelter	Volunteer to give free lessons related to your profession or hobby
Donate old clothes or household goods	Run or walk in a charity event
Volunteer at an animal rescue	Volunteer at a local museum
Donate to local food bank.	Serve a meal at a local shelter
Bring toys and stuffed animals to a children's hospital.	Volunteer at a local hospital
Send a care package or letter to deployed troops, veterans, or wounded soldiers.	Adopt-A-Family at the holidays

Table 5

Date Night Ideas	
Candlelight Dinner	Take an art class together
Bike Riding	Roller Blading
Progressive dinner: appetizer at one restaurant, main course at another, and dessert at a third location	Make your bedroom look like a hotel. Make hot chocolate, snuggle up and read to each other.
Treasure Hunt	Feed the ducks
Write down nice things you do for each other and read them out loud during dinner.	Get out old pictures of your life together and chat about your favorite memories.
Volunteer together at a soup kitchen or shelter	Swing on the swings at the park holding hands.
Write a song together	Plan a scavenger hunt
Take in a local sporting event	Attend a play, musical or concert together
Audit a class together	Make dinner together
Hike together	Visit Local Museums or Art Galleries
Ride a city bus or train for the entire route	Take a picnic to a park or scenic spot
Recreate your first date.	Rent a canoe or kayak
Read a book together	Drive-in movie
Lie under the stars and talk	Visit a museum or zoo
Play board games or cards together	Go dancing
Play the Newlywed game.	Play I spy
Walk through a local botanical garden while holding hands.	Ping pong
Amusement Park	Snowball fight
Play cards at the park	Snowman building
Pick berries at your local farm	Attend a lecture
Make dinner together	Bowling
Watch a sunset at a lake or beach	Go on a double date
Watch home movies together	Skiing
Hang out at a local bookstore	Sit on a dock and watch the boats
Watch airplanes take off or land	Ice skating
Rent a bicycle built for two	Take a dinner cruise
Go camping	Go to a jazz club
Go for a long drive out in the country	

Index

A

acceptance   156, 157, 186, 195
acid reflux   97, 106
ADAPT   66, 67, 226
ADHD   161, 240
aerobic   41, 103, 106, 107, 108, 133, 237, 238
air pollution   137, 245, 246
alcohol   60, 77, 82, 97, 178, 181, 182, 184, 205, 211, 212, 235
Alcohol   234, 235, 255
allergy   14, 88, 89, 90, 135, 136, 138
anger176, 177, 180, 195, 196, 210, 211, 212, 260
angioedema   90, 91
anticipation   125, 126, 127, 128, 242
apple   45, 57, 68, 69, 81, 88, 94
artificial sweeteners   87
asthma   27, 112, 135, 138
attention34, 40, 60, 95, 108, 112, 117, 123, 125, 144, 152, 157, 162, 165, 190, 191, 195, 197, 199, 200, 204, 206, 213, 215, 240, 242, 246
autoimmune diseases   6, 9, 10, 87, 88, 148, 180, 186
automation   40, 93

B

bananas   89
bike riding   126
biofeedback   112

blessings   195, 196, 197, 258
breakfast   40, 44, 58, 69, 74, 75, 93, 200, 228, 229, 231
breast cancer   196, 205

C

CADR   138
calories   54, 55, 56, 57, 58, 60, 63, 64, 65, 66, 67, 68, 69, 74, 75, 76, 80, 81, 82, 83, 94, 95, 97, 100, 101, 103, 105, 106
cancer   6, 8, 9, 87, 100, 105, 126, 129, 167, 168, 176, 186, 196, 204, 205, 207, 224, 225, 226, 234, 235, 237, 240, 243, 245, 254, 260
canker sores   119
carbohydrates   61, 224
celery   88
Celiac disease   126, 127
cereal   64, 74, 78, 229
children   14, 30, 31, 109, 116, 122, 124, 125, 139, 146, 152, 154, 155, 161, 162, 163, 171, 180, 181, 182, 187, 205, 221, 228, 229, 230, 232, 236, 244, 250, 258, 259, 267
cholesterol   6, 74, 106, 123, 139, 142, 143
cigarette   35, 137, 243
coffee   75, 122, 191, 194
colorings   87, 88, 90, 91, 136
community   3, 17, 34, 36, 137, 147, 154, 164, 166, 167, 168, 170, 178, 179, 194, 253

crab 90
creativity 40, 151, 188
cucumbers 88

D

dairy 136
debt 184, 185, 256
denial 180, 181
dental 93, 119, 241
diabetes 6, 7, 8, 9, 61, 72, 74,
142, 143, 151, 180, 186, 189, 228,
231, 233, 234, 238, 239, 243
diets 2, 17, 21, 54, 224, 225
dinner 19, 62, 64, 65, 68, 69,
70, 74, 85, 93, 95, 103, 116, 122,
163, 164, 198, 268
dirty dozen 88, 90
discipline 29, 32, 251
displacement 180
DNA 186, 238

E

eating healthy 54, 57, 93, 95
eczema 87, 88
eggs 74, 136
elliptical trainer 19, 41, 102,
103, 106, 204
emotions 172, 176, 177, 180,
193, 205, 246
exercise 1, 5, 6, 8, 14, 17, 18,
19, 20, 22, 26, 27, 31, 34, 40, 41,
44, 45, 48, 60, 92, 100, 102, 103,
105, 106, 107, 108, 109, 112, 116,
117, 118, 133, 134, 142, 150, 151,
152, 154, 157, 161, 171, 172, 179,
188, 191, 192, 199, 202, 204, 217,
224, 231, 235, 236, 237, 238, 239

F

Facebook 34, 67, 122, 151
family 9, 15, 19, 26, 31, 34,
35, 36, 44, 48, 67, 78, 86, 116, 117,
118, 123, 126, 134, 137, 141, 145,
147, 149, 150, 151, 152, 163, 164,

165, 166, 167, 168, 170, 171, 178,
182, 183, 184, 188, 191, 192, 194,
201, 219, 221, 251, 266, 267
fast food 85, 112, 230
fish 136
FitBit 55, 92, 132, 198
forgiveness 198, 209, 210,
211, 212, 260
Four Column Process 42, 217
friends 3, 9, 19, 31, 34, 35,
116, 118, 122, 123, 147, 149, 150,
151, 164, 165, 166, 167, 170, 178,
192, 194, 197, 219
fruits 6, 17, 62, 65, 72, 87, 88,
89, 226
frustration 176, 177, 194, 195, 196

G

Garmin 55, 132, 198
grapes 88
gratitude 194, 195, 196, 197,
198, 199, 200, 201, 202, 203, 258
grief 180, 181, 182, 183, 255
grievances 209, 210, 212
grocery store 44, 58, 72, 77,
87, 88, 166, 194

H

happiness 3, 4, 10, 38, 51,
100, 139, 195, 197, 199, 203, 213,
219, 246
Harvard 54, 111, 164, 245, 254, 257
Hashimoto's thyroiditis 88
healing111, 113, 178, 179, 181, 188,
205, 206, 213, 243, 248
healthy lifestyle 1, 2, 6, 8, 16,
17, 40, 51, 60, 92, 117, 142, 219,
237
heart 6, 8, 9, 10, 27, 59, 74,
87, 100, 112, 129, 131, 137, 139,
141, 154, 176, 177, 183, 184, 186,
189, 192, 198, 199, 201, 205, 206,
234, 237, 238, 240, 241, 244, 245,
253, 258, 261
heart disease6, 8, 9, 10, 100, 131, 137,

139, 154, 176, 234, 237, 238, 240, 241, 244, 258, 261
HEPA 137, 138
high blood pressure 6, 69, 72, 85, 97, 100, 118, 142, 180
hobbies 141, 142, 170, 205, 247

I

inflammation 57, 74, 87, 119, 127, 139, 180
inflammatory bowel, disease 87
Instagram 34
integration 39, 40, 45
integrity 186
Integrity 256
intimacy 158, 159

J

Jawbone 55, 132, 198
jealousy 176

K

kale 57, 63, 88
kindness 156, 157, 162, 168, 177
kitchen 44, 76, 77, 117, 146, 268

L

linkage 49, 101, 102
lobster 90
longevity 3, 4, 7, 8, 10, 17, 24, 27, 34, 38, 41, 57, 119, 126, 156, 158, 166, 167, 176, 178, 188, 191, 213, 219, 260
love 156, 158, 161, 164, 182
Love 250, 251, 252, 254, 255
lunch 47, 62, 67, 68, 69, 72, 74, 75, 78, 93, 94, 95, 118, 165, 197, 227

M

meaningful life 178, 188

medication 26
meditation 108, 109, 110, 111, 112, 113, 118, 133, 147, 181, 199, 200, 213, 240, 260, 261, 266
mentors 170, 171, 172, 173
minerals 59, 74
motivation 19, 40, 44, 101, 103, 189, 204, 231
mouthwash 90, 120, 127, 137
movies 18, 20, 21, 103, 151, 268
music 2, 49, 103, 139, 141, 151, 172, 201, 204, 205, 206, 207, 215, 247, 258, 259, 266

N

nectarines 88
nutrient-dense foods 57
nuts 136, 265

O

oatmeal 40, 57, 58, 62, 69, 74, 78, 93
observation 156, 157
one-hour rule 132
oranges 58, 59, 89
organic 88, 89, 232
osteopenia 106

P

pain 1, 37, 147, 167, 180, 181, 182, 183, 204, 205, 206, 209, 210, 211, 212, 239, 260
parenting 8, 124, 139, 161, 163, 170, 252
peaches 57, 88
peanuts 136
personal responsibility 32, 37
personal trainer 108
pesticide 88, 232
phytonutrients 61
Pilates 112, 133
portions 6, 7, 58, 82, 95
prayer 198, 199, 201, 254
present moment 181, 199, 213, 214

projection   180, 181
protein   6, 54, 65, 74, 75, 106,
   126, 224, 225, 264
psoriasis   87, 88, 182, 183, 186

R

reactivity   126
relationships   3, 6, 8, 17, 26, 31,
   37, 47, 60, 147, 156, 157, 158, 162,
   164, 165, 176, 186, 187, 188, 250,
   251, 252, 253, 254
Relationships   252, 253
Relaxation Response   111, 239
religion   178, 179, 198, 248
repression   180, 255
resentment   212
restaurant   45, 47, 55, 69, 80,
   81, 82, 84, 117, 184, 202, 230, 268
restless leg syndrome   133
rheumatoid arthritis   126

S

self-love   156
shellfish   90, 136
skiing   126
sleep   1, 6, 8, 16, 17, 26, 27, 31,
   55, 60, 83, 97, 100, 108, 112, 117,
   118, 120, 131, 132, 133, 134, 135,
   148, 151, 152, 154, 158, 159, 179,
   182, 184, 199, 204, 211, 212, 243,
   244, 258
sleep apnea   83, 133
smoking   129
Smoking   242, 243
snoring   83, 120, 131, 133, 159
social media   34, 48, 166, 201
soda   60
soy   136
spinach   57, 88
spiritual practice   171, 178, 179, 198
spirituality   8, 17, 178, 179, 254
Stanford   100, 154
steps   16, 19, 37, 38, 41, 66, 77,
   88, 89, 100, 101, 102, 103, 110,
   119, 126, 128, 134, 145, 147, 157,

198, 199, 236
strawberries   62, 88
stress   1, 6, 8, 17, 26, 27, 39, 46,
   60, 69, 100, 109, 112, 116, 117,
   126, 133, 134, 144, 146, 147, 148,
   154, 155, 157, 159, 161, 165, 176,
   179, 180, 182, 184, 185, 186, 188,
   195, 199, 205, 207, 240, 255, 258,
   260, 261
sugar   47, 55, 56, 57, 61, 71,
   74, 75, 77, 80, 82, 151, 152
supplements   25, 58, 59, 61,
   107, 127, 137
sweet bell peppers   88

T

teaching   10, 48, 161, 188, 189, 191
tomatoes   57, 88
toothpaste   90, 119, 120, 127, 137
Twitter   34, 201
two-hour rule   132

U

UCLA   1, 4, 58, 135, 221
ulcers   97

V

vacation   110, 111, 139, 144,
   148, 151, 199
vascular disease   87, 180
vegetables   6, 17, 61, 62, 65,
   72, 81, 87, 88, 89, 106, 226
vitamin   59, 107
vitamin D   107
volunteer   154, 155, 167, 267

W

watermelon   89
weight   5, 6, 9, 10, 33, 51, 54,
   55, 56, 58, 60, 65, 68, 69, 70, 74,
   75, 82, 83, 92, 93, 94, 95, 97, 100,
   101, 106, 107, 108, 117, 131, 151,
   224, 225, 226, 227, 228, 229, 231,

232, 233, 234, 235, 236, 237, 244, 250

wellness   1, 2, 3, 4, 7, 17, 23, 24, 26, 32, 34, 51, 54, 57, 93, 126, 140, 147, 149, 151, 166, 170, 180, 191, 217, 218, 219

wheat   136

whole grains   17, 74, 77

wine   97

wisdom   170, 171, 200, 201, 260

Withings   55, 92, 132, 198

X

xylitol   119, 120

Y

yellow No. 5   90, 91

yoga   106, 107, 109, 112, 133